the
new
meno
pause

ALSO BY MARY CLAIRE HAVER, MD

The Galveston Diet

Navigating Your Path Through Hormonal Change with Purpose, Power, and Facts

the new meno pause

Mary Claire Haver, MD

RODALE

NEW YORK

No book can replace the diagnostic expertise and medical advice of a trusted physician. Please be certain to consult with your doctor before making any decisions that affect your health, particularly if you suffer from any medical conditions or have any symptoms that may require treatment.

Published in the United States by Rodale Books, an imprint of Random House, a division of Penguin Random House LLC, New York.

rodalebooks.com

Rodale Books is a registered trademark, and the Circle colophon is a trademark of Penguin Random House LLC.

Library of Congress Cataloging-in-Publication Data has been applied for.

ISBN 978-0-593-79625-2
Ebook ISBN 978-0-593-79626-9

Printed in the United States of America

Book design by Elina Cohen
Watercolor background throughout by Shutterstock.com/Unchalee Khun
Floral leaves throughout by Shutterstock.com/lisima
Jacket design: Irene Ng

10 9 8 7 6 5 4 3 2 1

First Edition

TO MY CHILDREN KATHERINE AND MADELINE HAVER,
MAY YOUR MENOPAUSE TRANSITION LEAD TO THE MOST VIBRANT,
PRODUCTIVE, HEALTHY, AND BEST THIRD OF YOUR LIVES.

TO MY PATIENTS AND STUDENTS,
YOU INSPIRE ME EVERY DAY TO BE THE BEST MENOPAUSE
PROVIDER AND EDUCATOR I CAN BE.

Contents

Part Three: Symptoms and Solutions

Letter to the Reader

Dear Reader:

As a board-certified ob-gyn, I have spent countless hours in hospital rooms, in my clinic, in birthing centers, and in the operating room. In these spaces, I've heard the anguished cries of birthing mothers and brand-new babies, and details of confounding symptoms originating in and from the wildly complex and fascinating female reproductive system. I studied for years, endured grueling residency hours, and dedicated over twenty years to clinical practice so that my understanding of this system would allow me to support and engender women's health. I prided myself on my commitment to this specialty and on my ability to actively listen to patients.

Yet it wasn't until I began to be active on social media that I discovered that throngs of women had been yelling loudly for years, but no one had been listening. And they were desperate for help. These were women in perimenopause or menopause, and they felt isolated and distressed by a collection of disruptive symptoms. They often could not find support, from spouses or from friends; worst of all, doctors and other healthcare providers were denying them the legitimacy of their symptoms. Each woman seemed to feel isolated in her own dismay and despair.

I'll admit there was a time when I wouldn't have heard them either. But once I went through menopause myself, I *got it*. I could relate not just through empathy but through my own personal experience—I too had my life severely disrupted by sweat-soaked sleepless nights, annoying and unhealthy weight gain, frustrating brain fog, significant hair loss, and drying skin.

In my case, being on a birth control pill for contraception and to control my polycystic ovarian syndrome had likely staved off perimenopausal symptoms in my late thirties and early forties. When I was about age forty-eight, however, my healthcare provider and I decided I should stop taking the pill and "see where I was hormonally," knowing menopause was coming soon. Around the same time, my beloved brother, Bob, became terminally ill, and in my rush to provide him care at the end of his life, I forgot my own. I was devastated by Bob's death, and I attributed many of the physical and emotional symptoms I was having—most notably new belly fat and little sleep—to my grief.

I tried to be tough and power through it. But night after night of disrupted sleep changed my mind. I tried melatonin, meditation, and proper sleep hygiene, but nothing was working. The loss of sleep made me groggy and fatigued during the day, which made it harder for me to find the energy to exercise and easier to choose less healthy foods. It was a vicious circle of lethargy and unhealthiness! Finally, I decided to start hormone therapy, although for a number of reasons that I now know are common (and somewhat misguided), I felt as if doing so was an act of throwing in the towel.

I was lucky that I had the ability to self-diagnose and self-treat. I was also fortunate in that I had access to research and medical insight that helped me create a comprehensive approach to my own care. This included nutritional strategies, exercise, and stress reduction techniques. Fortunately, the combined approach worked, and I began to feel better. I can't overstate the profound relief I experienced when I started to feel like myself again.

Soon thereafter, I decided to share many facets of this approach in a program I created called the Galveston Diet. I offered this program first through my clinic in Galveston, Texas, and then later in a book of the same name. I began talking more and more about menopause on social media—and my reach has grown to over three and one-half million followers across my channels.

To say the response was overwhelming is an understatement. The program clearly spoke to and met a need that many had for a realistic and attainable approach to improving symptoms of perimenopause and menopause utilizing lifestyle and nutrition. I am so proud of the program and how many people it has helped and will continue to help.

But there are always more women to reach, to help. Indeed, the population entering this phase of their lives is not just big, it's *enormous*—by the year 2030, the world population of menopausal and postmenopausal women is projected to increase to 1.2 billion, with 47 million new entrants each year. Can you imagine the power of a population this size if we can unite to demand continued improvements in the standard of care for women at this stage of our lives? We could rally behind my personal mantra for *The New Menopause:* Menopause is inevitable; suffering is not.

Of course, even though we are in the midst of changing, this is a big ship to course-correct, and it's going to take a long time to get everyone on board and heading in the right direction. Yet simply by reading this book you are already on the gangplank; you have access to information and proven strategies that can help improve your quality of life and increase longevity.

So let me say this: I hear you. I see you. This book is for you and anyone else (partners, family, coworkers, supporters of any sort) seeking a better understanding of the menopausal transition and life after reproduction ends. My hope is that it will help educate and empower women to care for themselves or to help others care more deeply for them as they experience and deal with these changes.

A book may not be able to take the place of an in-person doctor's appointment, but the pages ahead present an opportunity for a fresh start in how you are or will experience perimenopause (the precursor to menopause), menopause, and postmenopause, and how you approach your well-being during these stages of life. Many will argue that menopause is a natural process and we should just let it take its course and allow our bodies to do what they're supposed to do. My response is that yes, the process is natural, but that doesn't mean that it is not harmful.

What do I mean by that?

Well, as your body naturally produces less estrogen (the hallmark of "the change"), your risks for developing serious medical conditions—

including diabetes, dementia, Alzheimer's, osteoporosis, and cardiovascular disease—go up. You may choose to change nothing about your lifestyle or hormonal levels to deal with the risks for these serious conditions, but I firmly believe that you should be fully informed about the range of those risks, as well as the options for mediating them. Put simply, perimenopause and menopause signal significant changes to your health, and you should be able to make an informed choice about the future of it. This book will put that agency in your hands, no one else's.

Mary Claire Haver

You'll see many stories from my patients and social media followers throughout this book. They're not the typical before and after stories you might expect. Rather, they are intended to demonstrate the many, sometimes surprising, ways menopause symptoms may manifest. My goal in providing these stories is to allow you to see what may be your own truth in the testimony of others and to validate you and your experience.

Part One:

THE STORY OF MENOPAUSAL MEDICINE

CHAPTER 1

It's Not All in Your Head

"We know our bodies; we know when something physically has changed."

"At age forty-seven, I was told by a gynecologist that perimenopause isn't real and was asked if I had a psychiatrist."

"I was told by my former doctor that women use menopause as an excuse to gain weight and that it's not real."

"I was told that it's all in your head."

"Welcome to your new normal."

"It's discouraging to not be taken seriously."

"Consulted my ob-gyn about perimenopause and mood swings, sexual interest. She blew me off and said I was too young for menopause."

"The migraines are a new symptom. I have only had them a few times, but they were debilitating. My doctor suggests I take Tylenol and lie down. I would prefer to address the cause and not just the symptom."

"Dr. said it wasn't perimenopause if I wasn't having hot flashes."

"I had to go to an ob-gyn and three cardiologists before I found one who believed me and had knowledge that it could be linked to hormonal changes."

"I was sent for a full blood screening and thyroid testing. All tests came back with good results, so my complaints were not addressed further."

"Still suffering."

That's just a small sampling of comments shared on my social media and in a research study on women's experiences with menopausal symptoms. The study, published in the *Journal of Women's Health* in 2023, sought to understand what kind of support a patient felt she was getting from her healthcare providers (and how that support could be improved). Overwhelmingly, the responses revealed substandard care and weak support. Many patients felt invalidated or reported that they hadn't been provided with any help or even given access to information that would allow them to understand the cause of their symptoms. My informal "survey" on my social media posts directed to gynecology patients revealed many of the same sentiments. Women said things like "My doctor told me he doesn't believe in perimenopause" and "I was told it's just a natural part of aging, get over it," and described encountering a medical attitude of "Welcome to your new normal." Sadly, these experiences aren't the exception, they are the rule. There are so many problems with this that I'm not even sure where to start. But first on the list is the fact that there are major medical consequences of this denial of care and guidance. If a woman in perimenopause or menopause is not getting top-notch care, it's a matter of life and death. Really.

Here's why: Your symptoms, of which dozens (including the well-known hot flashes and the not so well-known frozen shoulder), are the direct result of declining estrogen. My patients, colleagues, and I have been taken aback by the emerging research that's starting to explore the relationship between the menopausal drop in estrogen and issues like chronic cough, tinnitus, and benign position vertigo—just to name a few. These are issues that many women are attributing to "getting old" while they scramble to be believed, get help, and thrive during what should be a powerful and exciting time in their lives.

Estrogen isn't just a pretty hormone that's key to reproductive capabilities; it's responsible for so much more. There are estrogen receptors throughout almost every organ system in your body, and as your levels drop, these cells begin to lose their ability to assist in maintaining your health in other areas, including your heart, cognitive function, bone integrity, and blood sugar balance.

The list goes on, but in these areas alone we can spot a few diseases that regularly land in the top ten causes of death in women: heart disease, stroke, Alzheimer's disease, and type 2 diabetes. While osteoporosis isn't on this list, it still presents a serious concern, as one in two women will break a bone in their life because of bone loss from osteoporosis, and hip fractures alone are associated with a 15–20 percent increased mortality rate within one year of the break. All this is to say that estrogen is broadly and profoundly protective of your health, and its diminishing status during perimenopausal and menopausal years is a very big deal and should be treated as such.

In the pages to come, I'll present you with a head-to-toe tour of just what you can do to prioritize taking care of yourself during this *big deal* phase. Before we get to the strategies, I want to take a step back and establish some foundational understanding of the myriad ways that hormone changes can present themselves and why exactly the symptoms and resulting suffering have for so long been inadequately addressed.

Estrogen Replacement and Aging

If you are a candidate for hormone therapy, its use may prolong your life. A study published in the journal *Menopause* reported that a woman starting estrogen at fifty can expect to live up to two years longer than women who do not, and per year it's associated with a 20 to 50 percent decrease in dying from any cause.

So Many Symptoms, So Little Support

Stop me if you've heard this one before: A patient walks into a bar . . . or actually, it goes . . . a patient walks into their doctor's office first and *then* a bar after because they've been told, *yet again,* that the symptoms they've been experiencing for months, years even, are just normal or natural and associated with aging, that they're a manifestation of mood changes that just have to be endured, or, most insulting of all, that "it's all in your head." (No wonder the rates of alcohol use in women have climbed, although this is not a healthy trend.)

The not-so-funny reality is that you've likely not only heard it before but experienced it too. The question is: Why? Why can you go to a doctor seeking help, describe your symptom or symptoms, and then walk out feeling dismissed, absent a diagnosis, and without hope of any relief on the horizon?

In medicine, we look at this question in terms of access to care. That is, if there's an ideal patient experience, what are the barriers keeping people from having that kind of experience—the kind where a patient leaves a doctor's office feeling supported and empowered, and outfitted with treatment options? Let's take a look at the barriers to this kind of experience.

Lack of Awareness

One of the most significant issues responsible for inadequate treatment for those in the menopausal transition or in menopause is the insufficient understanding around its pathology, which is how an underlying condition or disease may present itself symptomatically. Changes in hormone levels can lead to a variety of symptoms that manifest in unique ways in each patient, making it difficult to recognize, diagnose, and treat.

It would serve physicians—and patients—well to get to know the list of potential symptoms because it extends far beyond hot flashes, night sweats, loss of bone density, and genitourinary symptoms. Here are many of the symptoms that may be related to perimenopause or menopause (see the Tool Kit for strategies to manage these symptoms).

Acid reflux/GERD	Bloating
Acne	Body composition changes/belly fat
Alcohol tolerance changes	Body odor
Anxiety	Brain fog
Arthralgia (joint pain)	Breast tenderness/soreness
Arthritis	Brittle nails
Asthma	Burning sensation in the mouth/tongue
Autoimmune disease (new or worsening)	Chronic fatigue syndrome

Crawling skin sensations

Decreased desire for sex

Dental problems

Depression

Difficulty concentrating

Dizzy spells

Dry or itchy eyes

Dry mouth

Dry skin

Eczema

Electric shock sensations

Fatigue

Fibromyalgia

Frozen shoulder

Genitourinary syndrome

Headaches

Heart palpitations

High cholesterol/high triglycerides

Hot flashes

Incontinence

Insulin resistance

Irritable bowel syndrome

Irritability

Itchy ears

Itchy skin

Kidney stones

Memory issues

Menstrual cycle changes

Mental health disorders

Migraines

Mood changes

Muscle aches

Night sweats

Nonalcoholic fatty liver disease

Osteoporosis

Pain with intercourse

Sarcopenia (muscle loss)

Sleep apnea

Sleep disturbances

Thinning hair (on head)

Thinning skin

Tingling extremities

Tinnitus

TMJ (temporomandibular disorder)

Unwanted hair growth (whiskers)

Urinary tract infections

Vaginal dryness

Vertigo

Weight gain

Wrinkles

Simply by looking at this list you can see how profoundly far-reaching hormonal changes can be, and how exactly an individual could visit nearly every medical specialty chasing a diagnosis if the common denominator of diminishing estrogen isn't identified. This is also why menopause symptoms may be mistaken for symptoms of other conditions, leading to misdiagnosis—or how it is possible to have more than one cause of similar symptoms (hypothyroidism and perimenopause).

Lack of Uniformity of Symptoms

Healthcare professionals love uniformity, and menopause is an out-of-the box nonconformist with highly individualized expression. Though the endocrine changes are relatively similar across individuals, the symptomatic experience can be distinct and diverse. Not all women will experience all of the symptoms I listed, but the majority will experience some. *When* a person has symptoms can vary too. Menopause symptoms can begin during perimenopause and can last for decades. You might be bombarded by multiple symptoms during perimenopause and reach smooth sailing during postmenopause, or experience the exact opposite.

We have a saying in medicine that if it walks like a duck and talks like a duck, it is a duck. Well, what kind of duck is menopause? It depends on the day, on the time of day even, and, as growing evidence shows, on a whole lot more. How menopause expresses itself in your body can depend upon genetics; lifestyle factors such as diet, exercise, smoking, and reproductive history; and influences like weight/BMI, climate, socioeconomic status, and even cultural beliefs and attitudes around menopause.

No Standardized Diagnostic Criteria or Screening

There is a medical definition for menopause: the point at which you have gone without a menstrual period for twelve months. But that means that you really only know you are "there" until that year has elapsed. Before then—as your periods become more sporadic (or sometimes heavier and more frequent)—you are in limbo, knowing that something is changing but unsure of how long the transition will take. That's the perimenopausal stage, but it's by definition *unpredictable*. I like to describe it as the "phase of chaos." And it has no universally accepted definition or specific diagnostic criteria; currently, there is no established one-time blood test that can tell your doctor where exactly you are in the process. A wide variety of changing symptoms means no specific and clear diagnosis for perimenopause.

There is also no routine screening of patients. In medicine, health screenings are used to detect the presence of a common condition or disease before symptoms appear so that prevention strategies and other actions can be taken to improve outcomes. We screen for high blood pressure; certain types of cancer, such as cervical, breast, and prostate; osteoporosis; depression; and more. Often these screenings are conducted using some type of tool or medical technology, but for some conditions, such as depression, the screening is done by having the patient complete a questionnaire.

There's no standard screening for perimenopause, in part because there's no cure or prevention for what's coming; menopause cannot be avoided. However, we know that many of the conditions or diseases that are initiated as you enter perimenopause and continue into postmenopause occur as a result of declining levels of estrogen and other sex hormones. Proper screening would not only alleviate symptoms and confusion but also allow for the implementation of targeted preventive steps that could lengthen both health and life span.

Gender Bias and Stereotyping

It's true that menopause affects only people who have female reproductive organs, but unfortunately, it is often viewed condescendingly as a "women's issue" and it is rarely taken seriously by doctors or our culture. As a result, very real life- and health-altering symptoms are dismissed as emotional and psychological in nature, or are categorically dismissed as mood swings that a patient should just tolerate or tough out. Unfortunately, this is not a new trend—in fact, it has been going on for thousands of years.

In Greek mythology, women who we now know were probably experiencing menopausal symptoms were described as having "uterine melancholy," or a distinct form of madness derived from their womb. Later, the Greek physician Hippocrates coined the term *hysteria* to refer to a vague disease also originating in the uterus, which he believed would wander around the body and cause symptoms such as tremors and anxiety through the release of toxic fumes. I wish I was making this stuff up. (If you want to know more about the history of women's health, check out the fantastic book *Unwell Women* by Elinor Cleghorn.)

Even though Hippocrates practiced medicine nearly 2,500 years ago, his theories still appear to infiltrate the minds of many in the medical field and influence how they practice medicine today. The inherited belief that a woman's medical issues are solely emotional or psychological in nature has especially strong staying power and contributes to what is today referred to as the "gender pain gap." This term describes the confounding reality that while women experience more chronic pain and more chronic conditions than men, their pain is more likely to be minimized and mistreated. If you are a person of color and a woman, you are doubly invisible and even less likely to get your pain treated properly.

This "gap" isn't just a theory; it's been proven to exist. Studies have shown that women who present with the same severity of pain as men in an emergency room wait on average sixteen minutes longer to get pain medication (if you've ever been in severe pain, you know that sixteen minutes is an eternity) and that women are more likely to be prescribed sedatives or antidepressants than pain meds. Women are also more likely to wait longer to be seen and to get less time to address their issues than male patients.

I hate to say it, but these stats come as no surprise to me. That's because I've seen this dismissive treatment firsthand, and at an early point in my medical career I was guilty of the same.

When I was in medical school, and then a new doctor in the 1990s, I was made aware of a patient type referred to simply as "WW." These patients would typically come in describing a cluster of symptoms: weight gain, brain fog, irritability, joint pain, decreased sex drive, poor sleep, and fatigue. "You've got a WW in exam room 3. Good luck with that," a colleague would say. This meant, and I cringe as I write this, that I was about to encounter a "whiny woman." Here we were practicing modern medicine, yet we were conflating legitimate symptoms with an emotion just like ancient physicians.

At the time, my colleagues and I knew it was likely that these patients were entering the menopause transition. But we had precious little instruction or education on the proper diagnosis, management, and treatment of it.

Further, we'd been taught that women tend to complain and somaticize symptoms because of dissatisfaction with life circumstances and stress. The "It's all in her head" medical mantra was very much alive and well. If she was found to be postmenopausal (again, confirmed by not having had a period in more than twelve months), we might offer menopause hormone therapy (MHT) and send her on her way (this was prior to the release of the WHI results in 2002). If she was transitioning into menopause, well, we offered nothing, insisting she had to go a full year without a period before we could intervene.

The result of this general lack of recognition and underdiagnosis of menopause symptoms no doubt caused women to suffer needlessly. This was a reality that I wasn't fully aware of until I was beset by symptoms myself. I experienced intense body aches, sweat-soaked sleepless nights, thinning hair, weight gain, and dulled cognitive abilities. These symptoms interfered greatly with my quality of life, rocked my confidence in my professional abilities, and made me realize that I was not practicing good menopause care.

When it became clear to me that my erratic and declining hormone levels were responsible for how I was feeling, I thought of the patients who had been where I was and had sought help from medical professionals but didn't get the support they needed. I felt guilty and ashamed to have been part of the problem back then.

The good news is that the medical care of the menopausal patient is improving, but its improvement will be limited unless we acknowledge and actively work on breaking down the significant barrier of gender bias. In fact, not acknowledging this bias would only perpetuate the gaslighting and further invalidate the experience of those who have walked into their doctors' offices or into the hospital hopeful that they would be helped, and who have walked out feeling worse, a pamphlet for antidepressants in hand.

Inadequate Training in Medical School and Residency

On the basis of what you just read, you might be thinking that doctors are to blame for the insufficient care and consistent misdiagnosis of those entering menopause or existing after it—and yes, they/we have some culpability, especially those who have denied or continue to deny the validity or severity of a patient's symptoms. But placing the blame solely on medical practitioners misses seeing the forest for the trees. There are much larger issues at play, specifically related to what medical students are taught in school and what education practicing physicians are required to complete to retain their licenses. We will never see better management of menopause without emphasis on better education.

Here's why education matters: the duck. You remember the duck, don't you? Doctors like a path to diagnosis that goes like this: Here are the symptoms; these symptoms align with diagnosis X, Y, or Z. When tests rule out X and Y, the issue must be Z. There's your duck: Z. (I'm not making light of the patient experience; for the sake of demonstration, I'm simply trying to simplify what can be a really lengthy, intensive process.)

A diagnosis is sometimes that simple, but not always, and there's nothing arbitrary about it. A doctor is practicing intellectual recall, drawing on years of study to attach symptoms to potential causes and following standard medical practice to produce confirmation because that's what doctors have been taught to do. But it turns out not many doctors have been taught how to practice medicine when it comes to the matter of menopause.

What is taught in medical schools and residency programs is limited in scope, showing only the most cliché symptoms of hormonal changes. What I learned in med school about obstetrics, general gynecology, pediatric gynecology, and gynecologic oncology and surgery was first-rate and important, but menopause got shoved in a box with "everything else" and received only a sliver of the time and attention. For example, in residency, I learned that menopause was marked by hot flashes, weight gain, mood swings, genitourinary symptoms, and sleep disturbances. That's it!

It took my real-life experience and hundreds of hours of self-driven research (i.e., it was not required for boards or to keep my medical license current) for me to understand that the presentation of endocrinological aging was so much more complex than those five common symptoms. I am an ob-gyn; my specialty is treating patients with ovaries, the two small, oval-shaped glands that produce estrogen, progesterone, and testosterone, the hormones essential to a menstrual cycle, fertility, and pregnancy. And it wasn't part of my required education to become more knowledgeable on the inevitable diminishing nature of this hormone production, or to understand its link to cardiovascular diseases, neurodegenerative disease, certain types of cancer, and lowered quality of life. I don't think that's right.

My training in obstetrics and gynecology began over twenty-six years ago, but unfortunately today's ob-gyn residents don't seem to be receiving much better education than I did on the subject of menopause medicine. A survey conducted in 2013 by researchers at Johns Hopkins found that nearly 80 percent of medical residents felt "barely comfortable" discussing or treating menopause. They also found that only 20 percent of ob-gyn residencies offered menopause training.

A later survey published in *Mayo Clinic Proceedings* revealed similar statistics collected from residents in obstetrics and gynecology, and in family and internal medicine as well. The residents who responded to this survey expressed a lack of confidence and competency in managing menopause and acknowledged a need and a desire for additional education— nearly 94 percent of respondents indicated it was important or very important to be trained to manage menopause.

When you consider these statistics, it's no surprise that most doctors don't know how to talk about, diagnose, or treat a patient properly during her menopausal journey. They're simply not being trained to do so. This is true even though one-third of American women are currently experiencing some stage of menopause and 51 percent of the population will go through this life-changing event if they live long enough.

If other doctors or medical school administrators are reading this, let me make my opinion and position clear: the medical community as a whole must treat menopause with the respect it merits, and that means prioritizing investments in curricula that teach today's up-and-coming doctors how to recognize and treat the menopause journey. For now, practicing physicians need to be proactive and seek out training from organizations such as the Menopause Society (formerly the North American Menopause Society), which offers continuing education courses and certifications in midlife medicine. We also need providers who do understand menopause to step up and help their fellow clinicians who need and desire guidance. Our patients deserve better care, and this will come in the form of recognition and validation of symptoms, and treatment of hormone depletion and the ensuing conditions.

An Insufficient Definition of Aging

One of the subtler reasons that women haven't received proper care for menopause is related to how the medical establishment defines aging as related mostly to chronological age (literally how old you are) instead of also considering a person's endocrinological age: the rate at which our ovaries age is twice as fast as for every other organ system in the body.

Like chronological aging, endocrine aging is inevitable, but unlike with most chronological aging, we have access to medical interventions that can restore hormone levels and help minimize the side effects of hormonal decline. The primary intervention is called hormone replacement therapy (HRT), also known as hormone therapy (HT) or menopausal hormone therapy (MHT). I prefer to use the term *MHT*. These are different names for the same approach, the goal of which is very straightforward: to replace or support the natural hormones that are no longer made by the body so as to help ensure that the functions initiated and promoted by these hormones are still conducted. You can think of it as a way of saying "Carry on with your work, heart cells, neurons, bladder cells, and joints."

I know the mention of hormone replacement therapy might bring up a lot of emotions, including fear. This is understandable—MHT has what some would describe as a troubled past, and it's not the right approach for everyone. But what I'm going to offer you in this book is something you maybe haven't gotten in your doctor's office, and something you deserve: a comprehensive discussion on the topic of hormone replacement therapy. You deserve to understand the truth about the research that scared so many away from MHT, and the emerging science that shows how safe and effective it may be in helping stave off the chronic diseases that start creeping in as estrogen declines. Not every person will choose hormone therapy, but everyone deserves an educated conversation. We'll get to that discussion in chapter 7.

There are other strategies, too, that can help support your body and mind during the menopausal transition and through to postmenopause. I'm excited to share them all with you and thrilled that you've put your trust in me to help guide you to feeling better and remain functional as long as possible. I hope you can benefit from what I've learned and unlearned about the best strategies and approaches. Together through awareness, education, and action we can be a part of the movement that clears the barriers to quality menopausal care. It starts here and now!

CHAPTER 2

The Complicated Past and Confusing Nature of Menopause Treatment

I officially entered menopause in October 2022 at the age of fifty-six. For the last year I have experienced terrible joint pain despite being at a normal weight, overall healthy, eating a healthful anti-inflammatory diet, and exercising several times a week. My primary care doctor did all sorts of labs including testing for inflammation and rheumatoid arthritis (all results were normal). My cholesterol was high for the first time in my life, and she told me to "continue working" on my already healthful diet. An orthopedic surgeon I saw about my joint pain told me I'm just "unlucky." Neither doctor ever put together that my joint pain or high cholesterol could have anything to do with menopause/lack of estrogen.

—Beverly W.

When it comes to biological brilliance, few things compare to the female reproductive system. This system is made up of a dependable team: the vagina, cervix, uterus, ovaries, fallopian tubes, and some ancillary, yet equally essential teammates that facilitate menstruation, support the development of a human being from embryo to newborn, and represent the parts of the anatomy that grant us the gift of sexual pleasure. Even twenty-five years after committing to the specialty of ob-gyn, I still marvel at its profound complexity, innate intelligence, and ability to perform seemingly superhuman feats of strength and endurance.

Consider the uterus: a small and hollow multilayered muscular organ that expands up to five hundred times its volume capacity during pregnancy. Or the ovaries: two almond-sized glands that at birth hold between one and two million oocytes, or eggs, which house all our unique genetic material.

These very same ovaries will produce hormones that regulate the menstrual cycle and maintain fertility, and they are the central organ in the production of estrogen. We owe much of our biological selves to estrogen; it's the hormone responsible for much of our reproductive tract, and it's important to the health of our breasts, skin, hair, heart and blood vessels, brain, and more. Estrogen levels fluctuate throughout our lives, rising and falling each time we menstruate, soaring during pregnancy, and, in healthy women, after puberty will be naturally suppressed or diminished during only two occurrences over our lifetime: postpartum and menopause.

Obviously, these examples demonstrate very different reasons for low estrogen: The first is to allow for lactation, the second is a result of what we in medicine call ovarian failure (sounds harsh, I know, but it is an accurate description of what is happening to our hormone production from the ovaries). But these occurrences bring about very similar metabolic changes. Yep, both breastfeeding moms and menopausal individuals can experience the joys of sleepless nights, hot flashes, dry vaginas, anxiety, and brain fog.

We know that these changes happen during lactation to prioritize the care of another living being. The lactating mother must wake often to nurse, radiate heat to warm a young infant, and be on alert.

When estrogen diminishes in the postreproductive phase, namely menopause, and all these symptoms arise, what's the point? There are some theories (see page 19), but I have my own suggested take on this transitional stage of our lives. I think we should consider these symptoms a sign that there's a living being needing great care. And that being is YOU. You need attention, you need love, you need support, and you should consider yourself ushered into an unprecedented era of much-needed self-care.

One problem is that there hasn't been a clear definition of what support and care look like during this time of great need. And if you're a patient, the doctor-recommended or prescribed treatments, if any are offered at all, have been inconsistent. In part, this is because the needs of the perimenopausal, menopausal, and postmenopausal person haven't been prioritized—not in society at large, and not in medicine, where women have long gotten less in the way of research prioritization and funding.

The treatments have also been inconsistent because our understanding of how to best manage the symptoms and lessen the health risks that arise during menopause has gone through so many dramatic swings and a trusted, foundational approach has not been established. This is so even though the answer has been there—or not there, as the case really is!—all along: estrogen.

It's important that we pause and look back at how we came to identify estrogen and its role in menopause, and how the medical knowledge of both has evolved over time. The past can teach us lessons about how we move forward and can help us create a better future for those who are next in line and will soon, when their own symptoms and health risks are rising in tandem, be asking: What can I do about this?

The History of the Mystery

The term *menopause* entered the world of words in 1821 thanks to the French physician Charles-Pierre-Louis de Gardanne. A mashup of *meno,* meaning "month" and relating to the moon, and *pause,* as in the stopping of something, the word quite literally means the end of your monthly cycle.

Long before there was a definition of menopause, it was a source of great confusion. Early Greek and Roman physicians thought the loss of blood via menstruation each month was a sort of purging of toxins and poisons from the body and that when menstruation ended in menopause, a failure to release these toxins would drive a woman mad. Over time, the approaches to treating this perceived "menopausal madness" would vary from wacky to inhumane and would include everything from using leeches to draw out toxins to locking women up in asylums.

Long Life After Menopause: A Head-Scratcher for Evolutionary Biologists

Given that the average life expectancy for women today is seventy-nine and the average age of menopause is fifty-one, women today can live at least thirty years past their ability to have children. We are one of very few animal species to have such a long postreproductive life span. This means we've basically hit the species jackpot, but it's also a fact that's puzzled evolutionary biologists who ask the question "How does menopause align with the survival of the fittest?"

The search for an answer has led some to theorize that menopause is an adaptation, introduced to allow women to live well past their reproductive capabilities so that they can help support and care for future generations, thereby enhancing genetic success; this is what's known as the "grandmother hypothesis." Other researchers believe that we are simply outliving our egg supplies thanks to our modern, civilized lifestyle. In other words, menopause is more like a modern luxury than a biological benefit that's helped advance our species in some way.

I suspect we'll never really know *why* we can live so many years past menopause, but I think from these theories we can glean a little bit for which we can be grateful. Most of all, we can be grateful for the fact that, in spite of the challenges that the menopausal transition can throw at us, we are fortunate to exist during an era in which we can live decades beyond the cessation of menstruation (and can do so more healthfully than ever before). This time represents an opportunity for us to create some of the best years of our lives. And guess who gets to decide whether *best* means dedicating our resources of experience, wisdom, and confidence to others who are younger than us, or celebrating the luxury of being liberated from our periods, or doing a little bit of both? YOU DO. Because whether it's thanks to evolution or not, you've earned it.

The treatments for menopause were so varied and ineffectual for so long because no one understood what was happening in the body (ovarian failure) to facilitate the end of a woman's cycle and, in most cases, bring about symptoms. It wasn't until the late 1800s and early 1900s that researchers began to zero in on the endocrine system, specifically the ovaries, and the existence of hormones as key to understanding the origins of menopause. It was around this time too that the first oral therapies, which were crude formulations of processed ovarian tissue from animals, were given in an attempt to try to help treat menopausal symptoms. Some of these treatments were shown promisingly to improve hot flashes and what was then referred to as "sexual dysfunction" (in modern medicine, we refer to it as hypoactive sexual desire disorder—low libido—or painful sex, both commonly experienced in menopause).

In 1923, American chemists Edgar Allen and Edward Doisy, the latter of whom would go on to win the Nobel Prize for his research on the chemical nature of vitamin K, became the first researchers to isolate a primary hormone produced by the ovaries. This hormone was determined to promote actions in the reproductive system related to a woman's cycle; they called it primary ovarian hormone. A few years later, it would become known by the name we all know so well—estrogen—the word being a combination of *estrus* and *gen*, as in the generation of a monthly cycle.

(Still with me? Just checking in to say that I know it would be easy to dismiss all this as dull historical detail. But these discoveries quite literally laid the foundation for our modern understanding of how the presence of estrogen influences menstruation and pregnancy, and how its relative absence introduces menopause. Read on.)

By 1933, estrogen was being manufactured and prescribed under the brand name Emmenin. It was produced first from extracts obtained from placentas, then from the urine of pregnant women, and it was used to treat dysmenorrhea, or pain associated with menstruation, and symptoms of menopause. Eventually it was reformulated from the urine of pregnant mares and was rebranded as Premarin, which the FDA first approved for the market in 1942. (It's important to note that there are now several hormone therapy options that do not rely on animals for production, and we will get into modern versions of hormone therapy in chapter 7.) Premarin's entrance into the hormone therapy arena would mark the start of a several decades' long seesaw of opinion and science related to hormone-based treatment for menopausal symptoms and related conditions.

The Rise and Fall and Rise Again of Hormone Replacement Therapy

Once it became apparent that there was a demand for ways to treat symptoms of menopause, drug makers got right to work. And in 1947, just five years after Premarin first got FDA approval, a total of fifty-three formulations sold by twenty-three different companies were on the market. Over the next couple of decades, sales of hormone replacement meds would continue to climb.

As interest in hormone therapy was growing, the national bestseller *Feminine Forever* was published. This book, written by the New York–based gynecologist Robert Wilson and published in 1968, promoted estrogen therapy as a way to preserve "femininity" and prevent disease. The book was influential despite being heavy on the ick factor, which you can spot right away in the tail end of the subtitle that says "Now almost every woman, regardless of age, can safely live a full sex life for her entire life." See what I mean? Ick. Not that every woman can't and shouldn't have a full sex life, but I don't think *Feminine Forever* was all about a woman's desire; the restoration of femininity promised by Wilson's book was promoted as a sort of "get your wife back" movement, and in this marketing, the priority was a man's desire and a woman's availability to fulfill it. *Ick.*

In any case, it *was* the sixties, and sex sells. Wilson's book definitely helped the sales of estrogen therapy. In 1975, estrogen formulations were the fifth most prescribed drugs in the United States, with thirty million prescriptions dispensed that year.

Then, in the last month of the very same year, other researchers published in the *New England Journal of Medicine* the results of their study on menopausal and postmenopausal women with a uterus, some of whom had been taking unopposed estrogen (that is, with no progesterone). When they compared those who had exposure to estrogen therapy to those who had not been taking estrogen, the former, they determined, had an increased risk of developing endometrial cancer. This prompted many women to stop taking estrogen therapy and led to estrogen-based products, such as MHT and birth control pills, being issued with new warnings about cancer risk.

Some Helpful MHT Definitions

In chapter 7, I will lay out all the details you need to help determine your MHT needs, including how to have a conversation with your own doctor (even one who may be dismissive or in the dark). For now, I want to introduce you to a few definitions:

Conjugated equine estrogens (CEE): a formulation made up of ten different types of estrogen, sourced from pregnant mare urine. Brand name: Premarin.

Medroxyprogesterone acetate (MPA): a synthetic progesterone (also known as a progestin) that is entirely lab produced. Brand name: Provera.

Other types of synthetic progestins include dydrogesterone, norethisterone, and levonorgestrel.

In the field of medicine, we are trained to consider whether the potential risks of a medication outweigh the expected benefits of a medication. In this case, the risks of malignancy in the endometrium were serious, yet the benefits were still there—reduced hot flashes and vaginal dryness, and a potential, promising link to preventing bone loss and osteoporosis. Work began to see if there was a way to lessen the risk of endometrial cancer, and evidence emerged that by adding a progestin, a form of progesterone, you could counteract the estrogen-induced changes in the endometrial lining. Prescriptions for this new combined therapy—estrogen and a progestin—

climbed, and by 1992, Prempro (conjugated equine estrogens and me-droxyprogesterone acetate) became one of the most frequently prescribed medications in the United States.

In the years that followed, research supporting the potential benefits of estrogen therapy began to be published, and influential organizations backed the use of MHT. The National Institutes of Health issued a statement that taking estrogen was the best way to prevent bone loss in menopausal women, and research showing a cardio-protective aspect of estrogen was building. Was it possible that hormone replacement therapy could prolong a woman's life? Some studies suggested that, yes, it was very likely this could be the case. One observational study showed 33 percent less fatal heart disease in women using estrogen therapy versus those who did not. The American College of Physicians proposed that all postmenopausal women, regardless of age or preexisting risk factors, consider MHT given its potential to prevent chronic disease. By the mid-1990s, 38 percent of women ages fifty to seventy-five were taking hormone replacement therapy. But soon the seesaw would shift again.

MHT Gets Put to the Test

There was a lot of good science coming out to support the general use of MHT, but it had yet to be tested by a randomized controlled trial (RCT), which is the gold standard of research methods. In an RCT, participants are assigned randomly to an experimental group or a control group. People in the experimental group get the medication or protocol being tested and those in the control group get a placebo, which is a fake treatment that appears real. Everyone in the study is under the impression they are taking the real thing, and all participants are treated and observed in identical fashion. This type of study is considered the best since it allows for researchers to get the most objective results possible (it's essentially the opposite of an opinion).

In 1998, the Women's Health Initiative (WHI) launched menopausal hormone therapy trials to finally use this gold standard of testing to evaluate MHT and its effect on cardiovascular disease and cancer in postmenopausal women. With twenty-seven thousand participants and a planned fifteen-year duration, it was part of the "largest women's health prevention study ever."

What happened next would again change the course of the use of hormone replacement therapy and alter the lives of an incalculable number of menopausal women. The outcome was so momentous that it deserves its own chapter, so keep reading!

CHAPTER 3

A Seismic Shift Occurs

I'm a clinical pharmacist who started my career just before WHI [the report on the Women's Health Initiative trials] was published. At the time, doctors refused to start HRT or stopped women from taking HRT. Patients were saying, "Don't you dare take my hormones away!" I couldn't comprehend why they were so vehemently against stopping. NOW, I UNDERSTAND. The little things I couldn't connect as perimenopause in my mid-late forties, I now know were all related. I was having anxiety and irritability that was way out of proportion to situations. I had hot flashes and insomnia for months without a break, which would wake me between 3:00 and 5:00 A.M. each morning and cause fatigue, daytime irritability, brain fog (for a pharmacist trying to make critical patient care decisions). I experienced joint pain, palpitations, sweating through clothes (while wearing a lab coat) and was uncomfortably hot all the time! I came to my last ob-gyn visit ready to argue for HRT. I was relieved when she said, "Let me help you." I still need a dose increase but I definitely see improvement. Don't you dare take my HRT away!

—Katie G.

When the Women's Health Initiative hormone therapy trials were first launched in 1998, I was in my last year of medical school at Louisiana State University Medical Center. By 2002, when the study was halted and the preliminary results were released, I was in my last months of ob-gyn residency at the University of Texas/Medical Branch. I remember vividly when the news came out. I was sitting in ob-gyn grand rounds and could hear my professors heatedly whispering about "breast cancer risks" and "calls from frantic patients." The study results had been shared via national news outlets before they were published. Patients were paying attention to the reports and calling their doctors in a panic. Practically overnight, 80 percent of prescriptions for hormone therapy were stopped nationwide, and from that point on, few new patients were offered the option of hormone therapy for their menopause symptoms. At the time, I had no idea that this memorable and momentous occasion would, years later, give me a new passion and purpose in my career.

The Women's Health Initiative (WHI) Study Design

There was a lot of optimism leading up to the WHI study around the use of MHT. Hormone therapy was known to relieve certain symptoms such as hot flashes and night sweats and was protective against osteoporosis and vaginal atrophy as part of the genitourinary syndrome of menopause (GSM). Multiple observational studies suggested that women on hormone therapy had a decreased risk of coronary artery disease and a lower risk of neurodegenerative diseases like dementia and Alzheimer's. This study, many thought, would produce the objective proof that hormone therapy was truly the standard of preventative care for postmenopausal bones, hearts, and minds.

I'm sure the fact that the study was going to happen *at all* generated a lot of excitement. Aging women were getting attention! And research funding! And time! It had taken researchers five years simply to recruit participants, and now even more time and money was going to be invested into the study of women in menopause. Simply arriving at the starting line felt like a huge win.

To make sure you have context, let's take a look at a few starting-line details. Who was there? Why were they there? Understanding some key points about how the study was set up will help the results make more sense.

The purpose: The Women's Health Initiative hormone therapy trials were designed to reveal the risks and benefits of hormone replacement therapy when taken by postmenopausal women with regard to the prevention of chronic diseases, such as cardiovascular disease and cancer.

The participants: The participants were divided into two groups: Group 1 consisted of 16,608 individuals with a uterus. Group 2 had 10,739 women without a uterus (due to hysterectomy).

The interventions: Group 1 was given estrogen and a progestin (to protect the endometrial lining in the uterus from cancer) or a placebo. Group 2 was given estrogen alone, also referred to as unopposed estrogen, or a placebo.

The duration: Researchers intended to follow participants for 8.5 years.

The outcome: In July of 2002, a follow-up with Group 1 revealed a slight increased risk of breast cancer. This group had also shown a *reduction* in incidence of colon cancer and osteoporosis-related fractures, but the breast cancer risks were prioritized and the part of the study looking at estrogen and progestin came to an early end.

Just a few years later, research on the second group, members of which had been taking estrogen only or a placebo, would also end early due to evidence of a small increased risk of stroke. Notably, the participants in this group did not present increased risk of breast cancer or heart disease, and they also showed lowered fracture and colon cancer rates.

The Results Heard Around the World

On the surface, this might seem like a very straightforward story with an unexpectedly dramatic outcome, but a deeper look shows that in reality it's very complex (and not so dramatic). Unfortunately, all the public got at the time was drama in the form of inaccurate reporting and alarming headlines, which—across the world—reduced the news to "estrogen causes breast cancer."

The media reinforced the message so repeatedly and so emphatically that the WHI study became the top medical story of 2002. The result, as I mentioned above: Women everywhere abruptly stopped taking hormone therapy, and 70 to 80 percent of those who had been taking hormones failed to renew their prescriptions. This means millions of women stopped getting relief from menopausal symptoms, and countless more failed to reap the preventative benefits of MHT.

I know the question you are asking in your head right now: *But what about the cancer risks?* Well, this is where the complexity comes in, and I'll do my best to respond with maximum clarity, because I know the risks associated with this study are very real (and I know the popular association between hormone therapy and cancer is as stubborn and resilient as a menopausal chin hair).

Getting Clear on the Risks of Hormone Therapy

The first thing to know about the results of the WHI study is that while the risks for breast cancer and stroke were there, they were not as significant or serious as initially reported, and they were most certainly overestimated and overemphasized by the media. Over the last twenty years, WHI investigators and others have come out publicly to clarify the data points on risk of cancer. And in 2018, the authors Avrum Bluming, M.D., and Carol Tavris published *Estrogen Matters,* one of the most important books on the subject of the WHI and the misinterpretation of the data that led to the erroneous reporting that estrogen caused breast cancer. Despite the availability of updated information, it has failed to get as much attention and the public opinion regarding MHT and significant health risks has largely remained unchanged. So I think it's time to give the details their due. Not everyone will want to read the level of detail I'll go into below. But I get questions about MHT and cancer risks every single day, and this is my chance to offer a thorough take on the science that planted this link in people's minds in the first place. To be clear, this isn't about convincing you that hormone therapy is right for you—that's a personal decision, and we'll go through the details in chapter 7—it's about providing greater clarity so that your decision is based on truth, not fear.

Below are some key factors in the WHI study that deserve a closer look:

Type of Risk (Statistically Speaking)

The focus of the reporting on the WHI study was *risk,* as in "women using hormone replacement therapy were seen to have an increased risk of breast cancer." What was never mentioned in the media was the type of risk being used to craft this message, despite the fact that type of risk matters a great deal—in fact, it completely changes the story of the WHI study.

The media often reports headlines based on what's referred to as relative risk rather than absolute risk, but the latter is what better represents the true risk. In order to come to a more accurate conclusion about the real risks of hormone therapy, we must consider the absolute value.

In the WHI study, the chance that a woman would develop breast cancer was four out of one thousand per year on placebo. When estrogen and progestin were added, that risk increased to five out of one thousand women per year. When this is calculated as relative risk, it's presented as a 25 percent increase. But when the data is instead calculated as absolute risk, the increase is 0.08 percent. In case it's not obvious, this is a big difference. A 25 percent increase is disruptive, it gets people talking. A 0.08 percent increase? Let's just say it would not have led to frantic whispers among my ob-gyn residency professors on that fateful day in 2002.

I want to point out here that the contemplation of risk types as it relates to MHT is not some fringe thing; far from it. In 2022, the Menopause Society statement on hormone therapy stated that "absolute risks are more useful to convey risks and benefits in the clinical setting." They also stressed the need for healthcare professionals caring for menopausal individuals to "understand the basic concepts of relative risk and absolute risk to communicate the potential benefits and risks of hormone therapy and other therapies."

I can tell you right now, simply on the basis of the number of comments and complaints I get over social media, that most physicians, including those offering healthcare to menopausal women, have not gotten this message. If they had, they would not still be categorically denying patients the option of hormone therapy because of its relative risk relationship to cancer.

It is also important to note that there was no increased risk of breast cancer during the first five years of treatment in any group.

What this means for you: Since 2002, reanalysis of the WHI data has led to the publication of hundreds of studies, many of which have acknowledged the inadequate reporting and the associated overestimation of risk that came from the initial review. Not even one of these studies has generated even half the attention that the original report did, and consequently the public and medical professional opinion on MHT has changed little in over twenty years. We must redefine, for patients and their doctors, the perception of risk associated with hormone replacement therapy. In many cases, the potential for benefits outweighs the risks, and every woman should be granted the discussion.

Drug Formulation

One of the significant flaws of the WHI study was the use of a single formulation of MHT. As you may recall, group 1 (the group associated with increased cancer risk) was given a combination of estrogen and a progestin. More specifically, the formulation was conjugated equine estrogens (CEE) and medroxyprogesterone acetate (MPA), which is a synthetic version of progesterone. Group 2 was given CEE alone; there was no increased cancer risk seen in this group.

This is significant for a couple of reasons. The first reason is that it's possible it was the type of progesterone used in the study that correlated to cancer risk and not the estrogen, as was reported. Again, the participants who took only estrogen saw no increased breast cancer risk; in fact, they actually saw a 30 percent lower risk than the placebo group. This suggests that estrogen alone may not promote cancer but instead protect against it—talk about flipping the script!

The other reason it's important to consider the drug formulation is that one form is not representative of all forms of MHT available, and some forms *may* be safer than others. Both CEE and MPA are types of hormone therapy and differ from the modern *bioidentical* options that are more typically offered today. MPA specifically is rarely used these days in MHT, as most informed doctors prefer progesterone such as that found in what doctors know as micronized progesterone capsules (Prometrium).

What this means for you: Not all hormone therapy formulations are the same. If you are considering MHT, see chapter 7 to review the available types (including what I mean by *bioidentical*), which differ based on how they are delivered to your body (e.g., through your skin [transdermally], through the mouth [orally], etc.), how they are produced, and what the evidence says as far as safety and efficacy.

Age When MHT Is Started (Timing/Healthy Cell Hypothesis)

Later analysis of the WHI data revealed a critical piece of information: The average age of participants in the study was sixty-three, much higher than fifty-one, the average age of menopause. The potential for this factor alone to negatively skew the results was very high. Older individuals are already more likely to have increased incidence of disease, including breast cancer and heart disease, with or without the introduction of therapeutic hormones, or any other medication for that matter. Younger women closer to the onset of their menopause were the ones most likely to benefit from the cardioprotective, neuroprotective, and musculoskeletal aspects of hormone replacement therapy. But these women *weren't* the primary subjects in the WHI study.

This realization grew into what's now referred to in scientific circles as the *timing hypothesis* or the *healthy cell hypothesis,* a theory that there is a critical therapeutic window during which the cardiovascular and overall health benefits of MHT can be optimized. The prime window of opportunity for cardiovascular disease is now believed to be within ten years of menopause, meaning if you were to begin using MHT before ten years had passed since your last period, the potential for benefits would be the greatest. And the benefits can be big: decreased death due to any cause and lowered instances of heart disease and heart attack. In general, the healthy cell hypothesis leads to the theory that estrogen is better at keeping a cell in a healthy state, and that the lack of estrogen leads to a cell being unhealthier—suggesting that estrogen may be better at prevention rather than cure. You will see examples of this throughout the book.

Of course, the whole purpose of the WHI study was to prove whether MHT was protective against the development of heart disease. And while initial review of the data suggested the effect was neutral, the timing hypothesis allows us to see the potential if, well, the timing is right.

For example, in the WHI study, in a subset of women ages fifty to fifty-nine, the risk of myocardial infarction (heart attack) in those using estrogen therapy was 40 percent lower than the risk among those who received placebo. On the other hand, MHT *initiated* by women ten or more years past menopause was associated with a slight but not statistically significant increased risk of cardiovascular disease, and with initiation of MHT after more than twenty years past menopause, the risk becomes statistically significant. What this shows is that estrogen therapy (through the action on nitric oxide formation) can make preexisting coronary artery disease worse. What we learn from this, courtesy of the American Heart Association (AHA), is that estrogen is better at preventing coronary artery disease than at stopping it once it gets started (the healthy cell hypothesis at work).

We need to take matters of the heart and women's health very seriously. Heart disease remains the number one killer in women, *even after a diagnosis of breast cancer,* and markers of declining heart health, such as dyslipidemia and increased arterial plaque, can be brought about by the loss of estrogen in menopause. The loss of estrogen signals a loss of resilience against those diseases. According to a groundbreaking statement issued by the AHA in 2020, the menopausal transition is *more of a factor than aging* in initiating "increases in lipids, metabolic syndrome risk, and vascular remodeling" (and this isn't the good kind of remodeling). Another reason why we should use the age of menopause to help determine an ideal candidate for hormone therapy: When it comes to heart health and MHT, the clock is ticking.

In the very same statement, the AHA referenced several studies that further demonstrate that early menopausal individuals may experience significant preventative benefits from MHT. In one example, researchers who had analyzed the results of nineteen randomized controlled trials found that women who initiated hormone therapy at or around age sixty (or less than ten years after menopause) reduced by roughly half their risk of cardiovascular disease.

What this means for you: If you are a candidate for hormone therapy, an increasing amount of science shows that MHT has the greatest potential to deliver preventative benefits when started less than ten years after your menopause. This means documenting the age at which you enter menopause is important, and so too is having the discussion on MHT with your *informed* healthcare provider (see chapter 8 for how to find a provider). The discussion doesn't have to wait—if you suspect you may be perimenopausal, the knowledge you gather now will not go to waste. See the Menopause Symptom Scoring Sheet in Appendix B to help determine whether the symptoms you are experiencing may be related to perimenopause.

Should ALL Women over the Age of 60 Avoid MHT?

When we look at the timing hypothesis, a critical question arises: Does hormone therapy after age sixty (or if you're more than ten years past menopause) do more harm than good? I know this question is especially relevant if you or someone you love fits this description.

My answer is that it depends. If a woman has been on MHT since early menopause and has not developed any increased risk factors for cardiovascular disease (such as an elevated coronary calcium test score, elevated ApoB, and/or uncontrolled hypertension), and she wants to continue, I will keep her on it, but I still think more research is needed in this area for this to have broader application. If a person is over the age of sixty or more than ten years postmenopause and has not used hormone therapy, the question of whether to introduce it is very nuanced and requires a detailed assessment of potential benefits and risks. In the benefits column, we have bone protection and reduction of genitourinary symptoms and hot flashes. As for the risks—there's a chance that if the person has existing coronary artery disease or is on the dementia spectrum, hormone therapy could contribute to the progression of these diseases rather than their prevention.

If I have a patient who is over the age of sixty or is in late menopause and has never used MHT, and has increased risk factors for coronary artery disease, I will have a coronary calcium score test performed (see page 75 for more on what this entails, and who should have it), check for a family history of Alzheimer's or dementia, and assess for general health. If the scan is low risk, she has no other significant risk factors for cardiovascular disease, there's no family history of neurodegenerative diseases, and overall health is good, only then will we have the discussion about starting hormone therapy.

You Deserve Better Than Outdated Medical Guidance

It's fair to wonder why, if there is so much science to support a rebranding of MHT, so many providers are still not offering it because they associate it with increased cancer risk. Well, as I've mentioned before, medicine is a slow-moving ship—it takes a very long time to course-correct—and this type of delay in the transfer of on-paper insight to real-life application is all too common.

A New Frontier for Fake "Cures" for Menopause

The news about the WHI study left many women too afraid to use the treatment they had been relying on to relieve symptoms of menopause and led them to start looking for alternatives. Who could blame them? Their symptoms were still there, even if the preferred treatment had been taken off the table, and they needed help. The demand for alternatives would open the marketplace to non-evidence-based approaches and would help usher in an era of questionable, even dangerous options being promoted as "cures" to menopause.

Before social media, you had to go out of your way to find alternative approaches. After social media, well . . . just try and hide from the ads promising a thirty- to forty-pound weight loss, a cured libido issue, or eliminated brain fog, all from just a vitamin, and let me know how it goes. Almost daily I get a message from a follower asking me: "Is this real?" Women are so eager for a solution that they will try almost anything, especially since they can't find support in the doctor's office.

So many products marketed as a cure/treatment for menopausal symptoms are *not* evidence based. See the Tool Kit for evidence-based strategies to manage your menopausal symptoms.

A big part of the problem is the failure to include significant ongoing education in the area of menopause in the board recertification process. Board recertification always requires a review—and proven understanding—of educational updates, but those that focus on menopause are simply not being prioritized—even in the area of ob-gyn, the medical specialty that focuses on women's reproductive system. I have a lot to say about this, but let's just say it's not fit to print.

Because the vast majority of ongoing medical education programs are not putting these articles right in front of doctors, doctors who want to become menopause "literate" have to seek out and interpret updated research on their own. And they have to do so in between back-to-back appointments while simultaneously completing corporate insurance paperwork demands, all while relying on a dwindling staff—and running off to deliver a baby and staying up all night on call. (It's not easy being a patient these days, but it's also a really tough time to be a doctor.)

This was certainly what life was like for me when I was a practicing ob-gyn. I struggled to keep up with all the menopause-related guidelines, yet the demand for menopause care was growing. The time came when I had to make a choice: Did I want to remain a physician who could focus on all aspects of women's health—pediatric gynecology, obstetrics, surgery, gynecologic oncology, *and* menopause—or did I want solely to focus on the postreproductive phase of life? The system wasn't and still isn't set up to allow a doctor to be successful in all these subspecialties that fall under the giant umbrella of women's health.

Ultimately, any physician who is going to promote themselves as a women's healthcare provider should know how to have an informed discussion on the topic of menopause. A discussion that fails to present an accurate portrayal of the pros and cons of MHT is not a discussion—it's a dead end, and women deserve better. But physicians too need better support and more focus on menopause in continuing medical education and research from the American Board of Obstetrics and Gynecology.

The good news is that today's medical trainees will be the first generation of medical residents to be taught that MHT is safe and should be discussed. Since it might take another generation before it becomes common practice, I encourage you to be a proactive patient. Who knows—you may have an opportunity to become the educator. On thepauselife.com, you can find links of current medical journal articles discussing the safety of MHT that you can print and share with your doctor.

CHAPTER 4

Together We Are Changing the Change

My menopause journey has taken me from a place of darkness to empowerment and hope thanks to increasing education. As a registered nurse for over thirty-five years, I was supposed to understand what menopause was about. But in reality, I was uneducated. I knew that frequent hot flashes were part of menopause, but I suffered so much more. Sleepless nights, painful muscles and joints, and heart palpitations prevented me from enjoying life. I was seen and treated frequently for UTIs, often only being reminded of how to maintain proper hygiene. I cried to my gynecologist when sex was so painful. The weight gain and redistribution was depressing, and my brain was foggy and I had difficulty finding my words. I honestly felt like I was dying. I'm happy to say that with education comes power!

—Sandy M.

A woefully small amount of research funding is directed toward women's health, and just a smidgen of this already miniscule amount gets invested in menopause research. In 2021, the National Institutes of Health reported that approximately $5 billion in federal funds in the United States was allocated for research in the area of women's health. Of this amount, research on menopause received a mere $15 million, which equals 0.003 percent of all federal funds for women's health research. Yeah, you read that right—menopause got less than half a percent.

This is the kind of stuff that makes me want to scream. This is not just meaningless behind-the-scenes, bureaucratic mismanagement of funds: The lack of funding directly affects the kind of care you will have access to during your menopausal transition and into your menopause. If you've had difficulty finding medical support and guidance, the problem can likely be traced back to these systemic deficiencies.

Thankfully, it makes others scream too, and the collective frustration is fueling collective action, helping to create a groundswell of change. We are witnessing unprecedented levels of corporate investment in menopause-focused research, medical technology, and product development. The tide *is* turning. Thanks to you and me and many amazing patients, physicians, thought leaders, and celebrities who are creating and pushing for change, we are finally getting some science and support to help reveal (or remind us of) the best and safest approaches to sustained health in the menopausal half of our lives. We still have far to go, and true change in the way we are cared for at this stage of our lives is going to take a long-haul commitment, not just the transitory interest of trend-hoppers eager to ride the menopause marketing wave (and reap financial benefit). But we are seeing promising signs of progress in the following realms.

Science and Research

For the longest time, little to no scientific research was being conducted on menopause. Then finally research was being done, but it was focused only on limited symptoms, such as menstrual irregularities, hot flashes, night sweats, and genitourinary symptoms, as well as health risks like diminished bone density. These are important areas of focus, but they really represent only the most obvious issues. Thankfully, modern science has broadened in scope, and researchers are now investigating many areas related to menopause, including treatment options, health risks and mood changes, cognition changes (brain fog), cardiovascular risk increase, insulin resistance/diabetes risk increase, musculoskeletal joint issues, and dermatological solutions. There is also a first-of-its-kind focus on how we define and treat the menopausal transition, aka perimenopause, because for some this time of life can be more mentally and physically tumultuous than postmenopause.

Influential groups are also helping to push progress. For example, the Menopause Society is promoting groundbreaking research in the area of menopause treatment and offering training and certification in menopause care. It is also continuing to provide and expand a helpful list of certified providers on its website (you'll want to vet menopause-certified providers; see page 123 for the questions I suggest you ask before you schedule an appointment).

The government is also getting legislative pressure to do more for menopause. A bill introduced in 2023 recommends that the NIH be required to evaluate the current state of menopause research, including identifying any gaps and calculating the total amount of funding the NIH has allocated for menopause and midlife women's health research for the previous five years.

Other medical societies, such as the American Heart Association (AHA), are recognizing the importance of the menopause transition and its role in worsening disease states, specifically with regard to cardiovascular disease risk. I mentioned (in the last chapter) the groundbreaking article published in 2020 by the AHA, which addressed the hormonal alterations that occur during midlife (or sooner) and highlighted their link to cardiometabolic health changes, such as increases in total cholesterol, LDL-C, and apolipoprotein B levels, that increase risk of heart disease. The AHA also acknowledged the cardioprotective benefits of estrogen and noted that the timing of when hormone therapy is started is likely relevant to the heart-related benefits. (Refer back to page 31 for more on the timing hypothesis.)

We are also starting to see the team of phenomenal researchers dedicated to the study of menopause grow. In the area of cognitive health, there are people such as Dr. Lisa Mosconi, who is an associate professor of neuroscience in the Departments of Neurology and Radiology at Weill Cornell Medicine, and the director of the Alzheimer's Prevention Program at WCM/New York–Presbyterian Hospital, and the author of the books *The XX Brain* and *The Menopause Brain*. Dr. Mosconi's work is focused on early detection and prevention of cognitive aging and Alzheimer's disease in at-risk individuals, especially women.

She has brought attention to a statistic that may be surprising to many, which is that two-thirds of all patients suffering from Alzheimer's disease are postmenopausal women. *Yikes.* Perhaps more unsettling than this is her remark that this discrepancy has for far too long been written off as inevitable simply because women live longer than men. In other words, it is often assumed that we should just accept this reality and move on. According to Dr. Mosconi, however, increased Alzheimer's in women is not a foregone conclusion or an unavoidable fate.

Her work, conducted with a team at Weill Cornell, has revealed that endocrine aging and the associated hormone changes, such as the precipitous decrease of estrogen during perimenopause and menopause, can accelerate chronological aging in the female brain. And this aging can equal increased risk of Alzheimer's disease as women undergo menopausal changes. While this might seem like bad news, it's actually positive because it suggests that there may be a time to introduce therapeutic interventions, such as hormone replacement therapy, to potentially help protect and preserve cognitive health.

Additional articles have shown the promise of early intervention. In January 2023, research published in *Alzheimer's Research and Therapy* showed that MHT had cognitive benefits in women with the APOE4 gene, carriers of which have a higher risk of developing Alzheimer's disease. Those who used hormone replacement therapy had improved delayed memory and larger volumes in brain areas important to information processing and memory when compared to nonusers.

This is all a "new frontier" kind of science that's focused on prioritizing prevention over acquiescence. We don't know for sure what protocols will work best in protecting the brains of women as they approach and enter menopause, but we know that people are working hard to figure it out.

In the area of ovarian health, people like Dr. Daisy Robinton, a molecular biologist with a PhD from Harvard University, are leading the way in groundbreaking ovarian research. Dr. Robinton is the CEO and cofounder of Oviva, a company working to develop methods to delay the decline of the ovaries and the negative health and quality-of-life consequences that come along with this.

Increased Access

I've heard from many people who have struggled to find a doctor or other healthcare practitioner to provide them with evidence-based menopausal treatment options, let alone acknowledge in the first place that their symptoms may be related to changes in estrogen brought about by perimenopause and menopause. The good news is that there are many more options now on the market, and I have no doubt that the access to quality menopausal healthcare will only continue to grow with time.

If you are looking for a physician or advanced provider to see for symptoms that you suspect may be due to perimenopause or menopause, you can start by visiting the Menopause Society's website to view their list of certified providers. I also maintain a list of providers who have been recommended by my followers at thepauselife.com.

If you discover shortcomings in medical support in your immediate area, one of the best workarounds is to give telemedicine a try and connect with a physician from a distance. There are some great companies that can help connect you with the right medical guidance, including Midi Health, Alloy Health, and Evernow. (I'm not sponsored by any of these companies; I just like what they are offering.) Of course, not every telemedicine option is going to be ideal, and for many women it's important to establish an in-person rapport with their doctor.

Product Options and Start-Up Opportunities

The number of products on the market to help address symptoms of menopause has exploded in recent years. It used to be that you couldn't find anything to help, but now you almost can't get away from ads featuring the newest, most promising product. There are products available now that claim to help with thinning hair, dry skin, painful sex, hormone balancing, and more. I'd like to say this is a quality problem to have—we now have the luxury of choice! But I recommend that you approach this choice with cautious optimism.

Even considering the recent increase in offerings in the menopause space, business insiders are acknowledging that there's still a lot more room for growth and are inviting others to get in on the innovation. This is good for us since competition will likely help push progress even faster and increase access.

Healthcare Cost Savings

I have heard so many personal stories from my patients and social media followers about the long and costly wild-goose chases they've been led on when trying to figure out the source of their symptoms. They've followed multiple referrals, made dozens of office visits (and paid the accumulating co-pays), and endured blood tests, heart checks, thyroid scans, and more. They have filled ineffective prescriptions, purchased pricey supplements, and bought countless boxes of Kleenex, which were needed to soak up the sobs when, after all their efforts, they were left with no clear diagnosis and no successful treatment options to speak of.

I know this is incredibly frustrating—but the future is holding more promise. As menopause education and access to care increase, more women will be told that what they're experiencing is likely the result of a perimenopause or menopause diagnosis, and they will hopefully be given all possible options of therapy, including hormone therapy.

Both of these developments will lead to a reduction of healthcare costs: first, because there won't be a need to see multiple doctors and run many pointless tests, and second, because women who are ultimately treated with hormone therapy have been shown to have significantly greater reduction in total healthcare costs after treatment initiation compared with untreated postmenopausal women.

The cost benefits will be seen too by those who need to address their symptoms with a non-MHT-based approach (yes, there really are other pharmacologic, over-the-counter, nutrition, and supplementation options to help with symptoms and promote health—I'll cover them all in the Tool Kit). Just getting to the answer that your hormones are to blame will help cut out diagnosis-chasing costs.

Workplace Support

Many women have reported that menopause disrupts their ability to work. In a 2019 survey of one thousand women over the age of forty-five conducted in the UK, symptoms such as hot flashes, low mood, trouble concentrating, memory challenges, increased depression and anxiety, and lessened self-confidence were noted as factors that contributed to making more mistakes, losing promotions, and even quitting a job altogether. Surveys conducted in the United States have reported similar conclusions, with one revealing that nearly one in five women have quit or considered quitting because of symptoms.

If you've worked through symptoms of perimenopause or menopause, I'm just telling you something you already know—that getting work done during this time of our lives can feel more grueling than ever. And this fact is made doubly difficult by the hard-to-shake feeling that you should keep the reasons for your distress to yourself; many who completed the surveys mentioned that they did not feel comfortable speaking to their employer or manager about their menopause symptoms and, in the United States at least, women said this was the case because they feared being discriminated against.

The answers provided by individuals here in the United States and across the pond gave clear proof that those of us in our menopausal years need more support from employers. When career and leadership coach Caroline Castrillon wrote about this topic for *Forbes* magazine, she had some smart suggestions on what that support could look like: menopause training for managers; access to menopausal resources; establishing a corporate menopause policy; and encouraging open conversations to help lessen the stigma that keeps so many women silent. Employees say they want flexibility that includes work-from-home options, temperature controls, and compassion and kindness (imagine that!).

It's in the corporate world's best interest to implement these kinds of changes since it's been estimated that menopause-related issues have contributed to productivity losses of over $150 billion globally. Some reports have shown that the number of employers offering menopause care benefits is increasing. Hopefully, since the bottom line is on the line, corporations will continue to step up and provide more support in the years ahead.

Media and Popular Culture:
Normalizing the Conversation

The explosion of social media over the past decade seems to have been a catalyst for women experiencing the symptoms of hormonal change to begin to openly share their experiences with more sympathetic listeners: one another. Unwilling to accept the status quo and suffer in silence, this generation of menopausal women is sharing symptoms, names of helpful healthcare providers, and functional strategies for navigating this time of their lives. They are arriving at medical appointments armed with research articles, lists, and resources to share with their providers so that they get the care they deserve.

Notable figures and celebrities such as Naomi Watts, Oprah Winfrey, Angelina Jolie, Michelle Obama, Viola Davis, Brooke Shields, and Salma Hayek are openly discussing their own menopause journeys, helping to lift the secrecy, shame, and taboo surrounding this time. Journalists, such as Susan Dominus with the *New York Times,* are writing articles that illuminate the topic of menopause, encouraging readers to question standards of care and demand better. Menopause specialists such as Dr. Louise Newson, Dr. Sharon Malone, Dr. Vonda Wright, Dr. Suzanne Gilberg-Lenz, and Dr. Heather Hirsch are writing books and leading important conversations on social media, and their followers are loving it, by the hundreds of thousands. When I turned to social media to discuss my own menopause journey, the conversation exploded into over three and one-half million TikTok, Instagram, YouTube, and Facebook followers eager to participate, share their stories, and ask for advice.

Together We Can Keep Progress Going

The progress that's being made is nothing short of amazing, but there is still much more to do. The outpouring of stories of frustration, misdiagnosis, gaslighting, and confusion have made many healthcare providers realize there is a systemic problem not only in how we provide basic care to a woman during her menopausal journey and how we teach and train our providers to care for these patients but also in how our society views and treats menopausal women in general. Together we can continue strengthening the foundation for the new future of menopause by:

- improving the education of our medical students, resident doctors, nurse practitioners, and physician assistants, as well as providing much-needed continuing medical education focusing on menopause care for our seasoned providers

- developing a deeper understanding about the physiologic processes of all phases of menopause

- learning how to advocate for ourselves

- sharing this book with younger women

- demanding new research and funding in the area of menopause

- increasing interest in and demand for more evidence-based treatment options

You've got this. You are not alone. You can't avoid this stage of life, so let's get through it together.

Part Two

GETTING TO KNOW MENOPAUSE (OR, EVERYTHING YOUR DOCTOR FORGOT TO MENTION ABOUT MENOPAUSE)

Despite the differences in how menopause can manifest in each person's life, some facts and definitions are useful for most women to understand, and in this section of the book I'm going to focus on these to help ensure we are all working from the same foundation of information. I like to think of this part of the book as a sort of stabilizing command center; whenever you find yourself asking, "What the heck is going on?" you can turn to these pages to gain some useful insight and, hopefully, comforting and helpful knowledge, the kind you can share with your friends and take to your doctor when you need to advocate for yourself.

The Three End Stages of Reproductive Change: Perimenopause, Menopause, and Postmenopause

I honestly thought I was losing my sanity. I knew about hot flashes/night sweats but nothing about the other symptoms. Lack of sleep due to night sweats, which caused me to be irritable and have anxiety and paranoid thoughts. I was becoming someone I did not like and was a little afraid of because I could not control my emotions or understand where they were coming from. But thankfully I now know that I am not crazy but normal. We talk about periods and sex education when we are younger—menopause should be included in that. Having the knowledge about what menopause is and being able to discuss it would have made going into it less traumatic for me (and no doubt for others, too).

—Susan P.

Ninety percent of women will approach their doctor with questions on how to cope with symptoms related to menopause. Many will walk away from their appointments without a diagnosis or suggested approach to feeling better, and then they will seek out resources online or elsewhere to offer some clarity. What I hope to provide in this chapter is a more concise and trusted version of this sought-after clarity. You'll find information that may help you better understand the menopausal landscape—and this is key, because even though it might feel like it, you are not walking on some foreign planet where no one has gone before; you are passing through a natural biological change, and I have the map to guide you through this journey.

The first critical piece of information to know is that the nomenclature around menopause can be confusing and misleading. Even though we call the entire passage "menopause" or call a woman "menopausal," in medical terms menopause is one day in a woman's life: the day exactly one year after her last period, and it represents the end of her reproductive function.

A woman's menopausal journey is made up of three discrete medical stages: perimenopause, menopause, and postmenopause. By definition, these are different stages, but in terms of experience they can feel very much the same. The reason symptoms can be similar throughout the stages of menopause is that they are all caused by deprivation of sex hormones (estrogen, testosterone, progesterone) that results from the decline and eventual end of ovarian function. It's usually the severity of symptoms, not the actual symptoms, that will vary as you move through the menopausal transition to menopause and then into postmenopause.

The duration of this entire transition will vary based on the individual, but research on women with reported hot flashes found that the average duration of symptomatic experience was nearly seven and a half years, and this average jumped up to almost twelve years in women who reported hot flashes earlier in their menopausal transition. It should be noted that these timelines are based on a limited understanding of menopausal symptoms and will likely evolve as more research is done and the science evolves.

While each person's experience may vary, some symptoms are more frequently experienced than others. One of the most reported symptoms has long been hot flashes, with or without the addition of night sweats, but I often wonder if it's the most common only because women know to connect it to menopause—they haven't been taught that the list of potential symptoms is much, much longer.

When Midi Health, a telehealth company focused on providing menopausal care, polled their twenty-two thousand members, the top five symptoms were weight gain/body composition change, brain fog/memory issues, anxiety/depression, sleep disruption, and hot flashes. My patients' most mentioned symptoms would also mirror most of these. As menopause education continues to reach a wider audience, my hope is that the understanding of the expansive expression of menopause will help an increasing number of women make the connection so that they are better empowered to seek support.

Can Any Test Diagnose Perimenopause?

There is no data that supports the use of any one-time blood, urine, or saliva test to definitively diagnose perimenopause; because our hormone levels at this time are wildly fluctuating, these tests are rarely informative or conclusive. Not even the DUTCH (Dried Urine Test for Comprehensive Hormones) test, a popular hormone test that generates results based on urinary metabolites, has been proven to confirm if you are in perimenopause or not. No data supports the legitimacy of this test, and no medical society recommends it.

However, the good news is there is a new serial form of urine testing that is showing promise as a way to diagnose early or late perimenopause. This urinary test requires five tests to be completed several days apart and comes with an app that collects a symptom profile and menstrual history. It generates a report that you can take to your physician that not only contains your results, but links to the medical evidence supporting the test results. Since so many clinicians are not menopause informed or trained, this test provides power to the patients.

Even without a diagnostic test, a good clinician who is menopause educated should be able to make the diagnosis of perimenopause by talking to you, *believing what you report to them,* and not automatically dismissing your concerns as related to aging or psychological issues. This doctor might also do blood work to rule out other diseases with similar symptoms, such as hypothyroidism, autoimmune disease, anemia, and others, and then begin planning your therapeutic course utilizing shared decision-making (making a decision with your doctor about your best course of action, after discussing your personal wants, needs, symptoms, risks, and benefits).

Now, let's look first at some of the distinguishing features of the menopausal stages, and then at what factors can influence your own menopausal timeline.

Perimenopause

Perimenopause is the beginning of the end of ovarian function. We often don't realize we are perimenopausal in the moment, but once through it, we can retrospectively pinpoint its beginning.

DEFINITION	Perimenopause is an extended transitional stage that happens before menopause. It is initiated by fluctuations in hormone levels, primarily estrogen and progesterone.
DISTINGUISHING FEATURE	Perimenopause is marked by irregular periods (longer or shorter in duration).
AVERAGE AGE	The entrance into perimenopause may begin in the forties or even in the midthirties.
AVERAGE DURATION	The data on this varies, but the average appears to be four years, with a range of two to ten years.

Perimenopause can be a challenging hormonal stage to diagnose. This is because (1) it has a wide range of symptoms and severity, (2) the age at which it presents itself in patients varies, and (3) there is no established method or evidence-based test for doctors to use to diagnose it. For these reasons, and for so many others that I've already mentioned—inadequate physician training and insufficient research funding, the long history of dismissive treatment of women, and so on—a physician may miss perimenopause altogether and send a patient down a medical rabbit hole trying to find a diagnosis for her symptoms. In fact, a survey of five thousand women conducted by Newson Health Research and Education found that a third of women wait at least three years for their symptoms to be correctly diagnosed as menopause related, and a further 18 percent visited their doctor six times before they got the help they needed.

When I have a patient who comes in struggling with symptoms that I suspect may be related to perimenopause, I follow a sort of clinical diagnosis tree (see following page) that helps eliminate other conditions that could be present. You can see in the "tree" how I might support a patient who came in with any of the symptoms listed at the top. The symptoms on the left, beginning with "hot flashes," are the ones we know MHT will help; the ones on the right are the ones we think MHT will help. Of course, I manage every patient on a case-by-case basis, but most often the questions asked to get to a diagnosis are the same. Because the hormone levels fluctuate so wildly in perimenopause, no one-time blood, urine, or saliva test can make the diagnosis. I make the diagnosis based on the patient's symptoms (and often do bloodwork to rule out other causes of those symptoms). In medicine, we call this a diagnosis of exclusion.

If you remember the duck from chapter 1, this is the work it takes to diagnose a person in any stage of menopause; it's a process that requires time, attention, and effort from your physician!

Menopausal Clinical Decision Tree
SYMPTOMS

Hot Flashes	Mental Health Changes
Night Sweats	Brain Fog
Menstrual Irregularities	Mood Disorders
Less Sexual Feelings	Sleep Disturbances
Visceral Fat Gain	Skin/Hair/Nail Changes
Painful Relations	Weight Gain
Genitourinary Symptoms	Muscle/Joint Pain
Hair Loss	Fatigue
Low Muscle Mass	Tinnitis/Vertigo
Bone Loss	Gastrointestinal Changes
	Burning Tongue

↓   ↓

**Evaluate Symptoms, Chronicity, Review Symptom Journal,
Sexual Function Screening**

Rule Out Overlapping Symptoms

Thyroid Evaluation	Restless Legs
Anemia Evaluation	Insomnia
Insulin Resistance Evaluation	Major Depressive Disorder
Nutritional Evaluation	Autoimmune Disease
Inflammation Markers	Alzheimer's Disease
Others as needed	

TREAT AS APPROPRIATE

 TREAT AS APPROPRIATE

Shared Decision Making

Hormone Therapy (Most Effective)	Hormone Therapy (Possibly Effective)
Nonhormonal Alternatives	Nonhormonal Alternatives
Nutrition Recommendations	Nutrition Recommendations
Exercise Recommendations	Exercise Recommendations
Supplemental Recommendations	Supplement Recommendations
Sleep Prioritization	Sleep Prioritization
Stress Reduction	Stress Reduction

Menopause

Though menopause has been the source of so much mystery, the event itself is the most clear and specific of the three stages.

DEFINITION   You reach menopause when it's been twelve months since your last period. This date will mark the end of your menstrual cycle and reproductive capabilities.

DISTINGUISHING FEATURE   Menopause is defined by a date on the calendar rather than specific signs or symptoms.

AVERAGE AGE	Average age of menopause is fifty-one, with normal menopause falling between forty-five and fifty-five years of age. Early menopause is defined as menopause that happens before age forty-five, and premature menopause before age forty.
AVERAGE DURATION	Menopause is one moment in time that happens when you've reached twelve months after your last period.

It's important to pay attention to your age as you transition into and eventually reach menopause because it's about so much more than just reproductive aging. Menopause initiates accelerated cellular aging and is associated with declines in general health. According to a 2020 statement issued by the American Heart Association, this is why a later age at natural menopause has been linked to longer life expectancy, higher bone mineral density and lower risk of fracture, and reduced heart disease. This makes sense when you consider the protective nature of estrogen; when it diminishes, there will be biological consequences. All the more reason to pay attention to changes in your menstrual cycle and any increase in symptoms that may be related to perimenopause, and to be proactive in treating these symptoms if they show up earlier than expected.

Postmenopause

It would be great if you passed into your full menopause and someone handed you some sort of reward for making it that far (I'd take a new set of cooling sheets that actually cool, please) . . . but all you get is, well, the prize of postmenopause. Postmenopause marks a turning point into a new stage of your life that lasts the rest of your life, one that potentially comes without the need to manage or plan around periods and offers an unexpected sort of freedom if you embrace it. My patients and followers tell me that now's the time your "give a sh*t factor" will decrease, and you will learn to set boundaries and prioritize yourself rather than your partner or children or job or parents or siblings. It's also a time when you should be kinder, more loving, and more giving toward yourself.

DEFINITION	You are postmenopausal once you've hit the menopausal moment—that is, when it's been more than twelve months since your last period.
DISTINGUISHING FEATURE	The highest prevalence of vasomotor symptoms, such as hot flashes, heart palpitations, and sweating, can occur in this stage, i.e., after the final menstrual period.
AVERAGE AGE	Postmenopause includes the rest of your life after menopause.
AVERAGE DURATION	Though you are postmenopausal for the rest of your life, common symptoms have been reported to last between 4.5 and 9.5 years after the final menstrual period.

Factors That Influence When You'll Enter Natural Menopause

There's no crystal ball that can predict exactly when you'll begin perimenopause or reach menopause (and therefore begin your postmenopausal stage of life), but there are factors that can influence the timing of these stages. Even though most of these factors are fixed—that is, you can't change them—knowing if you are high risk for an early menopause is important, as it can inspire action if it seems you may be more likely to enter early or premature menopause.

Genetics

Numerous studies have demonstrated that the primary influence on your age of menopause is family history. So if your mother or close relatives went into early, normal, or late menopause, your timeline may be similar. While your genes don't fully determine your menopausal fate, the odds are high that they'll play a big role.

Other research has found that the same genetic variants linked to late menopause are connected also to longer life, which further validates our understanding of how the endocrine aging that occurs during menopause can trip the switch on the systemic aging that follows.

Reproductive History and Menstrual Cycle Specifics

Women who have never birthed children are more likely to go into premature or early menopause compared with those who have. So too are those who had their first menstrual period at age eleven or younger. When these factors are combined, that is, someone has not birthed a child or children *and* they experienced menarche at a young age, there is a fivefold increased risk of premature menopause and a twofold increased risk of early menopause compared with women who started their periods at age twelve or older and had two or more children. Interestingly, the number of births may also influence how severe your menopausal symptoms are, with research showing that women with three or more births were more likely to have more extreme symptoms than those who had birthed one or two children.

Your cycle length can also influence your age of menopause. Specifically, individuals with a cycle length of less than twenty-six days may reach menopause close to a year and a half earlier than those with a longer cycle. Cycle irregularity, however, hasn't consistently shown to affect the timing of menopause.

It makes sense that your reproductive and menstrual cycle history can influence the timing of menopause. When you first start your period, you begin to ovulate, which is the process by which you release eggs from your finite supply (I'll go more into the details of this process in the next chapter). Barring an unnatural occurrence or disruption due to illness or some other health condition, you then ovulate once each month (or so) for about the next thirty-five years. If you started your period at an earlier age or you had more frequent periods, you are more likely to run through your egg supply, that is, reach menopause, at an earlier age. If you were pregnant one or more times, you skipped several months of ovulation (even longer if you breastfed) and retained those eggs that would otherwise have been ovulated, essentially delaying the onset of menopause. Despite this logic, it's important to remember that these aren't the only factors involved in menopausal timing.

Race/Ethnicity

In one study of age of menopause and ethnicity done in the United States, Native American and Black women entered menopause first, then non-Hispanic white women, and finally Japanese women. Some have theorized that the age differences in this study may be related to the genetic link to menopausal age, but it's difficult to isolate this from socioeconomic, life-style, and other societal factors that may also have varying degrees of influence on when you reach menopause. For example, when researchers analyzed data comparing the experience of menopause specifically between Black and white women, they found that elements of structural racism, defined by differences in access to health services and quality of care, contributed to disparities between the two groups in incidence of health conditions that predispose to earlier menopause and likely influenced the fact that Black women entered menopause 8.5 months earlier than white women. Black women also experienced more hot flashes and depression but were less likely to be offered treatment options.

We can't change the genetic influence on your menopausal timeline, but we can and we *must* work to overhaul the disparities that exist as a result of controllable factors by equalizing access to good menopausal healthcare, which includes the discussion of treatment options. This is more than a matter of making sure everyone has the opportunity to improve their quality of life in menopause; it's about potentially leveling the life span playing field. It's well established that greater incidence of hot flashes is linked to increased risk of dementia, stroke, and heart disease, which means Black women are set up to be disproportionately affected by these diseases. Thankfully, information and access are increasing with a focus on long-awaited and critically important inclusivity.

Weight and Body Mass

Research has shown that body weight can influence the age at which a woman experiences natural menopause. An elevated risk for early menopause has been seen in those who are underweight or have a low BMI in early adulthood or midlife, whereas later menopause has been seen in individuals with a higher weight or BMI. On the surface, this might suggest that more weight on your body can come with benefits since a later menopause can prolong your exposure to estrogen and its protective effects. However, too much excess weight, especially in and around the abdomen, may potentially counteract the benefits of delayed menopause and the associated hormone changes by driving up heart disease risk factors like lipid abnormalities (high cholesterol), blood sugar disturbances, and inflammation. So, what does all this mean? That being at a healthy weight— neither underweight nor obese—is what's most likely to benefit you in the areas of reproductive and overall health.

Premenopausal Cardiovascular Health

Having a heart disease event like a heart attack or stroke before the age of thirty-five doubles the chance of going through menopause earlier. This means that conditions like high cholesterol, high blood pressure, diabetes, and obesity can lead to early menopause rather than the other way around. One idea is that these risk factors cause a buildup of plaque in the arteries (atherosclerosis), reducing blood flow to the body. When blood flow to the ovaries is restricted, it damages the cells and tissues needed for reproductive hormones. This can speed up the process where follicles (egg-containing structures) don't develop properly, causing early menopause. In simpler terms, heart disease risk factors may contribute to early menopause by affecting blood flow and reproductive functions in the ovaries.

Physical Activity, Diet, and Alcohol Consumption

It's well established that regular exercise, a balanced diet, and limited to no alcohol intake are habits of good health, but can these lifestyle factors affect the age at which you enter menopause? There's no consistent science that says that they do, and really, we need a lot more research in this area. We do know, however, that these good habits can have huge benefits during peri- and postmenopause—I'll get into the details in the Tool Kit—and, given their relationship to heart health, can be holistically protective.

Cigarette Smoking

Research has confirmed a link between cigarette smoking and earlier age at menopause, with those who smoke being shown to enter menopause about a year earlier than nonsmokers. The longer the duration and the greater the intensity of a smoking habit, the greater the risk for premature or early menopause among current and former smokers.

History of Abuse

Research published in 2022 in the journal *Menopause* reported an alarming link between intergenerational abuse and age of menopause. The paper showed specifically that mothers who were physically abused and had a child who experienced regular sexual abuse reached menopause nearly nine years earlier than those without a history of abuse or abuse of their child. While there is no definitive conclusion yet on why this is the case, researchers believe it may be attributed to the cumulative impact of the body's response to trauma, which involves a routine flood of stress hormones that suppress the immune system and accelerate reproductive aging. As investigations on the effects of trauma continue, I expect we will only continue to see the devastating impact it can have on overall health.

Suppression of Ovulation with Oral Contraceptives

The ovaries contain immature eggs called oocytes that are recruited and essentially used up during ovulation. There's a theory that because the use of an oral contraceptive can reduce the recruitment of oocytes, it may delay menopause. This theory, referred to as the "oocyte sparing" hypothesis, has not generated enough scientific support to warrant the recommendation of oral contraceptives as a preventative against early menopause. However, there is some evidence that a woman's age when she starts using oral contraceptives may be relevant when it comes to potentially having an impact on menopausal timing. In at least two credible studies, researchers found that women who began taking oral contraceptives between the ages of twenty-five and thirty had a significantly lower risk of earlier menopause than women who were thirty-one years or older when they started.

Other Factors That Can Determine Your Menopause Timing

Some of us will lose our ovarian function before our time. This is usually due to surgical removal of the ovaries before natural menopause, chemotherapy or radiation for the treatment of a life-threatening disease, or premature ovarian insufficiency—we will discuss each in brief below, but they all lead to loss of our hormones before the natural expiration date—and this early loss of hormones accelerates certain associated symptoms and health risks.

Hysterectomy

Even if your ovaries are spared during a hysterectomy, the collateral blood flow to the ovaries is disrupted, and you can expect to enter menopause 4.4 years earlier than women without a hysterectomy.

Removal of One Ovary

There are a number of reasons you might need to have one or both of your ovaries surgically removed—an ovarian cyst or abscess or the presence of cancer, for instance. If you have both of your ovaries removed (bilateral oophorectomy, see below), you are effectively thrust immediately into menopause. Having one ovary removed is called a unilateral oophorectomy. If you have this done during your premenopausal years, it has been shown to accelerate the onset of menopause by 1.8 years. And the younger someone is when they have this procedure, the more significant the acceleration in the age of menopause may be. The loss of one ovary can bring about early menopause because you have a finite supply of eggs, and you lose half of whatever you have remaining when one ovary is removed.

Surgically Induced Menopause

Surgically induced menopause is abrupt, permanent menopause that's brought on by bilateral oophorectomy, or the surgical removal of both ovaries. You may have this procedure done as part of the treatment for ovarian cancer, for benign tumors, or for endometriosis. You may also elect to have a bilateral oophorectomy if you have inherited an increased risk for developing ovarian or breast cancer, or if you have gene mutations such as BRCA1 or BRCA2 or HNPCC.

Surgically induced menopause (surgical removal of the ovaries) is a big deal. It brings about sudden and dramatic changes in your hormones that can have severe consequences, if untreated, including introducing a 28 percent increase in overall mortality rate, a 33 percent increase in rates of heart disease, a 62 percent increase in risk of stroke, a 60 percent increase in risk of cognitive impairment, a 54 percent increase in mood disorder risk, and a 50 percent increase in risk of osteoporosis and bone fracture.

What this means is if you reach a state of disease or discomfort that may require the removal of your ovaries before menopause, you want to ensure that your doctor is certain this is the best and only course of action and that she has a plan to proactively and aggressively treat your menopause—especially if you are being offered an elective oophorectomy (removal of your healthy ovaries) during hysterectomy (removal of the uterus) as a purely preventative procedure. This is an outdated practice, and now we know that in most cases the health benefits of keeping your ovaries far outweigh the risk of a potential ovarian cancer. Of course, every patient scenario is unique, and you will want to ask directly: Do the benefits of removing my ovaries outweigh the risks? Certainly, if your life is on the line, the question answers itself. But other scenarios may be more nuanced, and you want to seriously consider your options before agreeing to a bilateral oophorectomy.

If you've had a bilateral oophorectomy or discover that you will need one before menopause, it's critical to discuss the option of hormone replacement therapy with your doctor. Studies show that hormone replacement therapy can eliminate the increased risk of cardiovascular disease in women with premenopausal bilateral oophorectomy, likely by slowing down the rate of atherosclerosis that accelerates with the sudden loss of estrogen that happens after your ovaries are removed. Research has also shown that when MHT is started within the first five years after menopause and is used for at least ten years, improvements in cognitive decline can be seen (more on this in chapter 6).

Chemically Induced Menopause

Chemically induced menopause can be caused by chemotherapy, radiation therapy, or hormone suppressive therapy. This type of menopause may be temporary or permanent depending on several factors, including your age, the intensity and duration of the treatment, and/or the type of drugs used.

Again, it's critical to discuss with your doctor the option of MHT and any other proactive alternative treatments to prevent the genitourinary syndrome of menopause (a group of symptoms and physical changes in the genitals and urinary tract that many women experience during and after menopause) and osteoporosis, and determine what options are available to you for the symptomatic treatments of hot flashes, night sweats, and sleep disruption. We will cover these in the Menopause Tool Kit.

Premature Ovarian Insufficiency (POI)

Premature ovarian insufficiency (POI) occurs when the ovaries stop working before the age of forty. You may hear this condition also be referred to as spontaneous or idiopathic POI or premature ovarian failure, but *insufficiency* is more accurate because if you have POI you may intermittently produce estrogen and ovulate, so it's not technically "failure." POI is caused by follicular depletion or dysfunction, and it can produce the same symptoms as menopause, including hot flashes and night sweats, painful sex, insomnia, mood swings, and melancholia. People diagnosed with POI can experience intense emotional and psychological symptoms, as these symptoms are often mixed in with the confusion and shock of needing to deal with chronic reproductive and hormone dysfunction before the age of forty. These feelings are exacerbated in women who receive a POI diagnosis after struggling to conceive a child.

There is still a lot of research that needs to be done before we fully understand what causes follicles to prematurely falter, but current science shows that POI may be a hereditary condition. It can also be brought about by:

- chemotherapy and radiation therapy

- autoimmune diseases, such as thyroid disease, Addison's disease, and rheumatoid arthritis

- genetic disorders, such as Turner syndrome or fragile X syndrome

- being born with a lower follicle count

- metabolic disorders

- exposure to toxins, such as cigarette smoke, chemicals, or pesticides

The reality of POI is that it causes a loss of estrogen and its protective effects at a young age. This can lead to an increased and earlier risk of heart disease, osteoporosis, and cognitive decline. It's critical for women with POI to find a supportive and proactive physician who can create a treatment plan that will help counter the significant health risks. An appropriate plan will include:

- hormone replacement therapy, if the patient is a candidate for it

- consistent exercise, preferably resistance training, to help combat muscle loss, a known consequence of POI

- psychological support, i.e., a referral to a therapist who specializes in infertility and matters related to reproductive health

- social support from support groups or online advocacy groups

- a consultation with an infertility doctor, if appropriate, to discuss pregnancy options, which may include the use of a donor egg

Even if you lose your ovarian function before your time, it's essential to remember that we are so much more than just our ovaries and the hormones they produce. You deserve as much prevention and anticipatory guidance as everyone else.

A Map of Menopause

Every person born as a woman will arrive at menopause one day. The paths we take may look different, but no one should ever feel lost. I hope that gaining an understanding of the stages of the menopausal transition and the factors that can influence the timing of your own journey have helped light the way.

CHAPTER 6

What Is Happening to Your Body During Menopause

I started with menopause symptoms around age fifty-two and stopped menstruating at age fifty-five. However, those three years were awful. I had symptoms that were so severe I saw a cardiologist, rheumatologist, gynecologist, and urologist. My male primary care physician wanted to put me on an antidepressant, and it definitely seemed like he knew nothing about menopause. I finally saw a menopause specialist and went on hormone replacement therapy, specifically an estradiol patch and oral progesterone. It truly saved my life. Within one week, I had no more hot flashes, night sweats, palpitations, or joint pain, and my mood swings got better, I had less fatigue and more energy, and my insomnia was gone. It has made my quality of life 1,000 percent better. Every woman deserves to know the truth about what the lack of estrogen does to your body. It's detrimental to our health when we lose it.

—Karen M.

Menopause evokes a lot of different emotions. Some women feel ecstatic at the thought of never having a period again—no more pads, tampons, PMS, cramps, or pregnancy risk! Others feel the exact opposite—they mourn the loss of their reproductive years, feel down about the clear sign of aging, and long to return to a younger stage of life. And then there are those who land more in the space of ambivalence. You know the person I'm talking about; she's the one who loves to say "It is what it is" way too often!

I hate to say it, but that friend who makes you roll your eyes or grit your teeth is right: It *is* what it is. Our bodies are finite and so too are our reproductive years; raging against this truth is futile. What is not futile is gaining an understanding of the changes happening in the body during perimenopause and menopause and then implementing actions and creating habits that will help protect you and potentially prolong your life in spite of these changes.

You don't need to know everything about menopause to get the support you need. But what will be helpful is to have a fairly detailed understanding of the changes in the endocrine system that lead up to menopause, as well as the significant impact these changes can have on the body. Many practitioners will use the difficulty of the subject and the general lack of knowledge to sweep your symptoms under the rug quickly without offering any potential solutions.

I've heard countless stories of basically the same patient experience, which goes something like this: You go to your ob-gyn with new and disruptive symptoms of what is most likely perimenopause. This doctor took great care of you throughout your reproductive years, performing Pap smears, issuing contraception, perhaps supporting you through pregnancy and birth, then maybe a surgery or two. But the symptoms that have brought you into the office this time don't get the same type of care, and instead you get dismissed and told there is nothing they can do to help you; you'll just have to be tough and power through it. Since you're still symptomatic, you find an alternative practitioner who is kind and listens to you, but instead of diagnosing your perimenopause—the duck—they diagnose you with adrenal fatigue, parasitic infestations, vitamin deficiencies, subclinical thyroid conditions, a buildup of toxins, or more! And you are given a supplement regimen or "detox system" that promises to balance your hormones for the price of at least a couple hundred dollars a month. It's not that vitamin deficiencies and subclinical thyroid conditions aren't real, but they are rare and more often than not are misdiagnoses. So hundreds or thousands of dollars later and still experiencing symptoms, you feel worse because you don't feel better and you begin to gaslight yourself—*It must be all in my head.*

If this hasn't been your experience, be thankful. Unfortunately, it is incredibly common.

So, what can we do to make sure you don't have this experience or at the very least you don't have it again? We can work together, and for my part, I can help ensure that you have access to essential information. Information is the foot you shove in the door before another doctor shuts you out in your search for answers. Use what you learn here to advocate for yourself and make an informed choice on what is best for your body during your menopause journey.

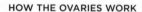

HOW THE OVARIES WORK

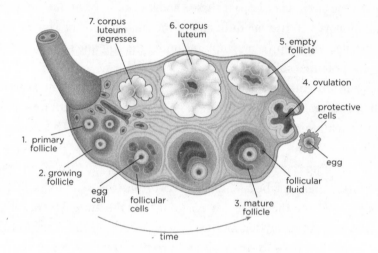

The Ovaries

Ovaries are almond-shaped glands. You're born with two of them, and they come prestocked with your lifetime supply of oocytes, or immature eggs, which usually equals between one and two million eggs. By the time you reach puberty, this supply has dwindled to between three hundred thousand to four hundred thousand oocytes. These little oocytes will rest within fluid-filled sacs called follicles until they are recruited during the menstrual cycle and potentially called up to be the dominant follicle of the month.

Phases of the Menstrual Cycle

The menstrual cycle is made up of four phases that prepare the body for pregnancy each month: menses, the follicular phase, ovulation, and the luteal phase. The whole process is wildly complex and, like a symphony, requires many different players to play each note perfectly in order for the performance to be a success (see chart below for a visual portrayal). Understanding how this process works in your reproductive years can help you better identify what's happening as you enter perimenopause and eventually your postreproductive years.

HORMONE LEVELS ACCORDING TO MENSTRUAL CYCLE PHASE

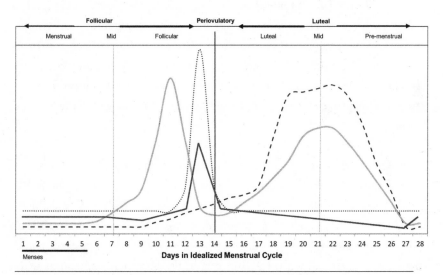

Draper CF, Duisters K, Weger B, et al. Menstrual cycle rhythmicity: metabolic patterns in healthy women. Science Reports 2018;8:14568. doi: 10.1038/s41598-018-32647-0.

1. Menses (days 1–5): The menstrual cycle begins with getting your period, which is the body's system for shedding the tissue, blood, and mucus that make up your thickened uterine lining each month. Menstruation is a sign that last month's ovulation has not resulted in pregnancy, and since your levels of estrogen and progesterone are not needed to help prepare your body for pregnancy, they will drop accordingly during this first phase.

2. Follicular phase (days 6–14): Now your body begins the process of readying you for pregnancy again. The ovaries release estrogen to help thicken the lining of the uterus, which will be needed if you become pregnant. Then the pituitary gland will release follicle-stimulating hormone (FSH) to trigger the follicles within the ovaries to begin to grow. Only a certain group of follicles will grow, and just one among this group (unless twins are on order) will emerge as the dominant follicle that will grow into an ovum, or mature egg. Specific cells in the follicle called granulosa and theca cells help drive growth by secreting estrogen and testosterone.

3. Ovulation (day 14 or so): An increase in a hormone known as luteinizing hormone (LH)—thanks again to the pituitary gland—will trigger your dominant follicle to release the mature egg in the process known as ovulation. The empty follicle will then collapse in on itself and form a corpus luteum, meaning yellow body. This temporary gland will produce estrogen and progesterone to help further the thickening of the uterine lining.

4. Luteal phase (days 15–28): The mature egg makes its way through one of your fallopian tubes and down to the uterus, where it may be fertilized by sperm. If the egg is fertilized and implants in the sticky and thickened uterine wall, you become pregnant. If this doesn't happen, the cells of the corpus luteum begin to disintegrate and levels of progesterone and estrogen drop to allow for the thinning of the uterine lining and, shortly thereafter, the menses phase again. The lowering of hormones at this time can produce symptoms of premenstrual syndrome (PMS).

This elaborate, incredible feedback cycle will continue this way for about thirty to thirty-five years unless you become pregnant or experience a disrupted cycle from disease or another health condition.

How the Ovaries Stop Working

As you age chronologically, you also age reproductively. As you menstruate and ovulate over this time, you progressively lose follicles, and with each new year your eggs lose quality. Your ovaries' functional capabilities begin to wane too, resulting in less reliable hormone production and decreased responsiveness to hormone signals. This decline in function will continue, causing disruptions in your cycle and creating symptoms of hormone withdrawal, which can signal the entry into the menopausal transition, aka perimenopause, and lead to irregular periods, hot flashes, increased anxiety, heart palpitations, and more.

The sped-up version of what happens next is this: The decline in ovarian function will continue, menstrual cycle disruptions may increase and lengthen, your symptoms may intensify, and so on until you reach ovarian failure. When you reach ovarian failure, the routine monthly ovulations and the resulting production of sex hormones will stop for good. And with the cessation of ovarian function, you will have reached menopause.

Of course, in the slowed-down version it's not nearly this straightforward. There is so much going on hormonally as your reproductive system starts to shift into retirement that it's really too detailed to cover in these pages. But I think getting a general idea of the hormonal havoc that's taking place can help remove some of the mystery around the symptomatic experience of menopause. This "(No More) Flow Chart" demonstrates the progression.

- Hormone fluctuations all start when your ovaries begin to run out of eggs. Fewer eggs means fewer follicular cells that surround them, and this equals decreased production of estrogen, progesterone, and some testosterone.

- The hypothalamus, a region of the brain that controls hormone production, senses the lower levels of estrogen in the bloodstream and responds by releasing more gonadotropin-releasing hormone (GnRH).

- This hormone, in turn, stimulates the pituitary gland to produce more follicle-stimulating hormone (FSH) and luteinizing hormone (LH) to help promote follicle growth and ovulation.

- If levels of estrogen and progesterone remain low, as they do if your ovarian function is declining, levels of FSH and LH will continue to increase (this is kind of like when you keep calling someone hoping they will pick up: *I know they're there, why aren't they answering?*).

- Your body is trying to find a way to generate estrogen, but it's running out of options. The number of follicles in the ovaries continues to decrease, and the remaining ones become less and less responsive to stimulating hormones as they age.

- Dramatic drops in estrogen bring on hot flashes and skipped ovulations, and other unpredictable symptoms arise.

The Truth About "Estrogen Dominance" and "Hormone Imbalance"

Some practitioners in the integrative medicine field use the terms *estrogen dominance* or *hormone imbalance* to oversimplify what's going on when you have unpredictable ovulation or other symptoms. They use this terminology because hormone fluctuations, even those that occur during a healthy menstrual cycle, are complicated and not easily explained. But understand this: Your estrogen levels are *not* elevated, as the term may imply. Instead, they are not "opposed" by the counterbalance of progesterone. Another way to say this? Your estrogen production is high *relative to* progesterone. It's also important to note that *estrogen dominance* and *hormone imbalance* are not terms recognized or used by all medical professionals. They are often too vague and imprecise to qualify for use in a clinical diagnosis or to allow for a doctor to create a treatment plan, and they are not indicative of the root cause of the problem.

If you were to come into my office with symptoms suggestive of a hormonal disorder or imbalance, the list of potential diagnoses could include polycystic ovary syndrome (PCOS), endometriosis, thyroid disorder, menopause, and more. And I would explore the potential causes of genetic predisposition, environmental and/or lifestyle factors, and reproductive aging (in the case of menopause). In each case, I would work with you to rule out underlying medical conditions. Never would I suggest you had a simple case of hormonal imbalance.

I know this might be confusing given the outrageous number of products and services out there being marketed as cures for hormone imbalance and symptoms such as fatigue, weight gain, mood swings, and low libido. The truth is that the majority of these products are not regulated, and their claims and promises don't have to be backed by medical studies; most, if not all, are likely to be ineffective and expensive, and there's the risk they could even be unsafe. I recommend staying away and instead finding a menopause-trained provider who will help you navigate this issue.

The Health Risks of Menopause

As I've said before, even though the loss of ovarian function and potentially uncomfortable symptoms that can accompany menopause (symptoms that we will address in Part Three) are *natural,* these aren't the only "side effects" of ovarian failure that require your attention; menopause, regardless of whether you have symptoms or not, puts you at increased risk for a daunting list of conditions and diseases. Your risk begins to go up as your estrogen levels go down (and these risks are added to the risks of aging that may already be present).

Estrogen is an incredibly protective hormone, and when it diminishes in menopause, we lose much of this protection. With estrogen out of the picture, stress hormones, such as cortisol, and other proinflammatory actors become more active and destructive—so much so that some researchers have labeled the menopausal transition as an "inflammatory event." This event establishes an internal trend toward chronic systemic inflammation, which can affect many organ systems and is a significant factor in the increase in health risks that comes with menopause. As a result of menopause, you are at increased risk for:

- osteoporosis

- coronary artery disease

- insulin resistance and prediabetes

- neuroinflammation

- visceral fat gain

- sarcopenia (loss of muscle mass)

I'm thinking primarily of this list of serious issues when I stress the importance of having a discussion on hormone replacement therapy with your doctor. Estrogen replacement therapy can have a preventative impact in these conditions. Yes, the symptom control is what may bring you to the point of considering MHT, but the broader health implications should be just as, if not more, compelling a reason to find out if you're a candidate for it.

Let's take a closer look at each of these conditions.

Osteoporosis

Osteoporosis is a progressive bone disease characterized by brittle, weak bones.

Your bone strength and mass naturally degrade over time, but when you are young, your body works hard to routinely fight the degradation, renewing your bones' strength and maintaining their mass. As you age, this renewal slows but the degeneration does not, and you can ultimately develop osteoporosis, especially if other risk factors are present. Having osteoporosis makes you more susceptible to bone fractures and breaks in the hip, spine, or wrist. These injuries are inconveniences when you are young but can be debilitating and dangerous when you are older. Hip fractures are especially concerning—research published in the *Journal of Internal Medicine* found that one in three adults aged sixty-five and over dies within twelve months of suffering a hip fracture.

Women are four times as likely to develop osteoporosis as men, and the loss of estrogen in menopause is the most common cause. This is because estrogen performs the important role of slowing the breakdown of bone. There are estrogen receptors in bone tissue, and they need estrogen to tell them to activate formation and increase production. When our estrogen levels plummet in menopause, osteoporotic bone loss is increased and bone weakness can result. Between 40 and 50 percent of postmenopausal women will experience a fracture related to osteoporosis during their life-times. Studies have also found associations between vasomotor symptoms, such as hot flashes and night sweats, and lower bone mineral density, os-teoporosis, and even bone fractures.

KNOW YOUR RISKS

There are several steps you can take to help prevent osteoporosis or pro-tect yourself if you develop this serious bone disease. The most important step is to get screened for osteoporosis if you've previously had a fracture in the hip, vertebrae, shoulder, pelvis, or wrist, or you have any other risk factor. Some of the key risk factors include petite body frame (weighing 125 pounds or less); early menopause; a history of smoking and/or heavy drinking (defined as two or more drinks per day); daily use of corticoste-roids, thyroid medication, warfarin, or other immunosuppressive drugs; bariatric surgery; and certain chronic medical conditions, such as kidney failure, rheumatoid arthritis, and liver disease.

KNOW YOUR NUMBERS

The most common screening test for osteoporosis is a bone density or DEXA scan. Most insurance plans will begin covering this screening at age sixty-five. However, if you identify with one or more of the risk fac-tors mentioned above, you may qualify for early screening. And even if your insurance won't cover the cost, I highly recommend getting the test done and paying for it out of pocket (the cost is between $200 and $300). (An added bonus to a DEXA scan: It measures muscle mass and visceral fat as well—see the section on visceral fat gain on page 81). If you have diminished bone density, the sooner you identify it, the better, as this will allow you to take proactive steps to slow bone loss and protect yourself against fracture. A bone fracture can be so debilitating and costly that you want to avoid it if at all possible!

HOW MHT MAY HELP

I will cover prevention and therapeutic strategies for osteoporosis in the Tool Kit, but it's worth noting that hormone replacement therapy has been shown to help protect skeletal health through menopause. Research published in 2021 reported that estrogen therapy may help prevent bone loss and reduce the risk of fracture by 20–40 percent, and its protective effect seems to have the greatest potential if it's begun within the first ten years after menopause. Furthermore, testosterone therapy may also play a role as our serum testosterone levels have been positively correlated to bone mineral density in perimenopausal and early menopausal women (we need more research in this area). In the next chapter, I'll discuss how to determine if you are a candidate for MHT and how to have a conversation with your doctor.

Coronary Artery Disease

Coronary artery disease is a specific type of cardiovascular disease that occurs when plaque made up of cholesterol and fats builds up in the arteries, reducing the flow of oxygen-rich blood to the heart. Reduced blood flow can cause damage to heart function and increase your risk for blood clots and heart attack.

Coronary artery disease is the leading cause of death for women, and our risk for developing it increases around age fifty-five, the age at which most women are already, or are soon to be, postmenopausal. The overlap in increased risk and timing of menopause is not coincidental, as menopause is known to drive up total cholesterol, LDL, and triglycerides, which are established risk factors for heart disease. (If you were surprised by a jump in your cholesterol levels during the menopausal transition, you're not alone!)

During menopause, there is also a concerning collection of changes that can occur in response to decreasing levels of estrogen and progesterone and that negatively affect your blood vessel function. When estrogen and progesterone diminish, blood vessels constrict more; your liver begins producing too much of the proteins that coagulate blood, increasing chances for blood clots; and endothelial cells, which line the blood vessels, make less of the hormones that help your vascular system relax and allow for smooth blood flow. These factors combine to create a serious threat to heart health.

KNOW YOUR RISKS

You may be at increased risk of coronary artery disease if you:

- have a family history of heart disease

- have high cholesterol, diabetes, or high blood pressure

- are a current or former smoker or have had long-term exposure to secondhand smoke

- have prolonged exposure to air pollution or other environmental toxins

- are overweight or obese

- are physically inactive

There are also factors related to menopause that have been linked to increased risk. If you experienced menopause before age forty-five, you are at significantly higher risk of developing heart disease when compared with women who went into menopause at age forty-five or later. Your risk is greater too if you experienced surgical menopause or if you have or had severe menopause-related symptoms, such as hot flashes and night sweats.

KNOW YOUR NUMBERS

What's most concerning about coronary artery disease is that (1) it doesn't often produce symptoms until it causes a rupture or becomes severe enough to block blood flow, and (2) there aren't really any great screening tests in place. That's not to say there aren't screenings in place at all: An annual physical will include checking your blood pressure, weight, and cholesterol levels, all factors that when high can increase heart disease risk.

They're just not *great* screening tests because they don't provide a detailed picture of what's going on in your arteries. A better test is a coronary calcium score test, which is a CT scan that looks at the level of calcium or plaque buildup that may be present in your coronary arteries. A coronary calcium score test reveals the presence or risk of coronary artery disease.

If you are over forty and considering using MHT for the first time, and you have significant elevated risk factors for coronary artery disease, I believe it's important to have a coronary calcium score test done prior to starting any medications. If your insurance won't cover it, I would consider paying out of pocket.

HOW MHT MAY HELP

Hormone replacement therapy has been shown to significantly reduce cardiovascular disease and death from all causes when used by women younger than sixty years old who are at or near menopause (no more than ten years removed from menopause). On the other hand, if MHT is started later than ten years after menopause, there *may* be an increased risk of cardiovascular disease, and that risk jumps even higher if it's been more than twenty years. This remarkable divergence is part of the timing hypothesis, which suggests that when you begin hormone therapy makes all the difference (refer back to page 31 in chapter 3 to read more on this). The key takeaway is that MHT appears to work best when used as a preventative tool in many diseases, but especially cardiovascular disease.

Insulin Resistance

Insulin is a hormone your pancreas makes that allows your cells to use the food you eat as fuel; it's about as essential as it gets when it comes to metabolic function and basically keeps the engine of your body running. When in its peak form, your metabolism will look a little something like this:

- You eat food, and your stomach and small intestines convert it to glucose (blood sugar).

- Your pancreas releases insulin to signal to your cells to use the glucose as fuel.

- Your cells get the signal and let in the fuel to be used, clearing glucose from the bloodstream.

- Your pancreas stops making insulin until the next time you eat or drink something.

This entire process can be disrupted if your cells become less sensitive to insulin, which is what happens if the condition of insulin resistance develops. In insulin resistance, the body's cells become less responsive to insulin, leading to high blood sugar levels. If blood sugar levels remain high for an extended period of time, this can lead to chronic low-grade inflammation.

I like to say that insulin resistance is the first stop on a train of metabolic dysfunction, which is why we need to take it seriously. If left unchecked, insulin resistance will put you at risk of reaching prediabetes and then type 2 diabetes. Insulin resistance is also what we call a gateway to metabolic syndrome, a group of conditions that significantly increase your risk of not just type 2 diabetes but coronary artery disease and stroke as well. Metabolic syndrome can include elevated blood glucose levels, elevated triglycerides, low high-density lipoprotein (HDL) cholesterol, and high blood pressure.

Because our estrogen levels decline during the menopausal transition, we are more susceptible to developing insulin resistance. Estrogen plays an important role in glucose metabolism, and its absence can contribute to metabolic dysfunction. The risk for insulin resistance due to declining estrogen is independent of age, meaning that even younger women who go into early menopause may be at risk of developing insulin resistance.

Believe it or not, I think insulin resistance represents a unique opportunity for metabolic correction; it is much easier to restore insulin sensitivity at this metabolic "station" before the more serious conditions of prediabetes and type 2 diabetes develop.

KNOW YOUR RISKS

Abdominal obesity (visceral fat) and physical inactivity are key risk factors for developing insulin resistance. You are also at increased risk if you have polycystic ovarian syndrome (PCOS), sleep apnea, or fatty liver disease. Some medications, including certain blood pressure medications, steroids, and those used to treat psychiatric disorders or HIV can make you more likely to become insulin resistant. Conditions such as Cushing's disease and hypothyroidism can also increase your risk.

KNOW YOUR NUMBERS

Your standard annual blood panel won't reveal if insulin resistance is present, and early symptoms may not be obvious. However, if your pancreas has reached a point where it needs to start pumping out more insulin in response to insulin resistance and if insulin levels remain high, you can develop high triglycerides and high blood pressure. If you have either of these and/or low HDL cholesterol, you have one or more features of metabolic syndrome, and high levels of insulin are likely. In this case, you want to be vigilant about getting your blood sugar levels checked. In my practice, I will evaluate a fasting glucose and a hemoglobin A1C on all patients, and if certain risk factors are present, I test fasting insulin and calculate a HOMA-IR score and then proceed. Homeostatic model assessment for insulin resistance (HOMA-IR) is a score that is calculated from a fasting insulin and glucose level. If you think you may be at risk for insulin resistance, I advise you to advocate for yourself and ask your doctor to run this test.

HOW MHT MAY HELP

While the research in this area is still developing, recent studies have shown that estrogen therapy may have a protective effect against insulin resistance in postmenopausal women. Additional science has found that women on hormone therapy had a 20 percent lower incidence of type 2 diabetes compared to those who were not using MHT. However, I still think we need more research before we can broadly use MHT for the specific purpose of reducing insulin resistance and other metabolic disorders. Until then, it's incredibly important to work on reversing or reducing the risk of insulin resistance with lifestyle strategies. I always start my patients with nutrition and exercise, the specifics of which I will discuss in the Tool Kit.

Neuroinflammation

Neuroinflammation is inflammation that occurs in the brain or spinal cord, and it can damage nerve cells essential to cognitive function. When neuroinflammation becomes chronic, the repeat damage can tangle up your brain's communication lines and potentially lead to the formation of the kind of plaque that's associated with Alzheimer's.

Women are twice as likely as men to develop Alzheimer's, which has long been attributed to the fact that women live longer than men and the risk of Alzheimer's increases as we age. But emerging research has found another contributing factor: the dramatic hormone changes we experience during the menopausal transition. These changes, especially the loss of estrogen, can increase neuroinflammation and, according to neuroscientist Dr. Lisa Mosconi—director of the Women's Brain Initiative and of the Alzheimer's Prevention Program at Weill Cornell Medicine/New York-Presbyterian Hospital—accelerate the chronological aging in the female brain. It's this aging that can equal increased risk of Alzheimer's disease as women undergo menopause.

It's possible that estrogen decline is also the reason why we are disproportionately affected by other cognitive-related diseases and disorders, such as multiple sclerosis (the autoimmune disease that attacks the brain and spinal cord), migraines, and major depressive disorder.

KNOW YOUR RISKS

You are at increased risk of neuroinflammation if you have high blood pressure, high cholesterol, heart disease, and/or type 2 diabetes. These conditions are proinflammatory and can directly compromise the health of your heart and blood vessels, which are responsible for transporting essential oxygen to your brain.

Your risk for Alzheimer's disease specifically increases as you age and if you have had a sibling or parent diagnosed with the disease. Latinx and African Americans also have a higher risk of developing Alzheimer's.

KNOW YOUR NUMBERS

Nearly everyone who goes through the menopausal transition will experience an uptick in inflammation, including in the area of the brain. This is an inevitable consequence of the decline of estrogen, which I've already pointed out plays a crucial role in regulating inflammation. Estrogen also is essential to managing certain neurological functions. It's no wonder then that menopause can affect clarity of thought, concentration, calmness, and other brain-related abilities and behaviors.

Unfortunately, there aren't any approved or effective tests to check for neuroinflammation. But we can sort of nonscientifically measure our cognitive response to diminishing levels of estrogen by paying attention to the severity of brain-related symptoms of menopause. This can include symptoms like brain fog and forgetfulness, and anxiety and depression. Most women will experience some of these symptoms, to varying degrees. "This isn't surprising when you think about how many menopausal symptoms—including hot flashes, depression, anxiety, sleep disturbances, and even brain fog—actually stem from the brain rather than the ovaries," says Dr. Mosconi.

Generally, the symptoms will get better as estrogen stabilizes, and you'll establish a kind of postmenopausal norm (it's unlikely that you will ever return to a premenopausal status quo). However, for some women, there will be a progression in the area of cognitive decline that may eventually lead to the diagnosis of dementia.

If you are at increased risk of Alzheimer's or other cognitive disease, I highly recommend that you read *The XX Brain* and *The Menopause Brain*, by Dr. Mosconi. She's an incredible resource for all matters related to menopause and cognitive health.

HOW MHT MAY HELP

There has yet to be a sweeping study saying that MHT is brain-protective for *all* women who are in or approaching menopause. But some research shows that it is effective for specific groups and not recommended for others.

As I mentioned in chapter 4, research published in 2023 found that carriers of the APOE4 gene, which is associated with a higher risk of developing Alzheimer's disease, experienced improved memory recall speed and larger volumes in brain areas when taking hormone replacement therapy (when compared to nonusers).

Hormone therapy has also been shown to be significantly neuroprotective when used by women who had a bilateral oophorectomy (removal of both ovaries) prior to the age of fifty, and somewhat protective in those who used MHT in the early menopausal stage, which is generally between the ages of fifty and sixty. However, women who began MHT in late menopause, defined as between sixty-five and seventy-nine, were shown to have increased risk of cognitive decline and dementia. This shows that, as with cardioprotection, the timing of MHT may be an important factor in determining whether it will be safe and/or effective for brain cells.

Visceral Fat Gain

Most women who are approaching menopause or have passed it undergo body composition changes. These changes are driven by the preferential weight gain of visceral fat in the deep abdominal region and may become noticeable when your favorite clothing items begin to feel tight or uncomfortable, or your body starts to seem unfamiliar (suddenly your pear shape has turned into an apple). This "shape shift" may happen even if your weight hasn't gone up significantly.

One of the main reasons people visit my office is this unwelcomed and often unexpected change. Women often come in feeling completely distressed, complaining that other healthcare providers offered only, if anything at all, vague advice to "work out more and eat less." My approach is to explain that a successful strategy will be much more specific than that, and I also stress the dangers of doing nothing to counter the effects of visceral fat gain. To be clear, I am not discouraging acceptance of your changing body—you should accept the heck out of your body and all it's done for you! But that doesn't mean you should acquiesce to changes that can have serious health consequences. Let's take a look at how the gain of visceral fat can affect your health.

There are basically two types of abdominal fat. There's subcutaneous fat, which is the type of belly fat that exists more on the surface that you can pinch. This fat, regardless of how you feel about it, is relatively benign from a health perspective as long as you don't have too much of it. Then, there's visceral fat. Visceral fat is a type of belly fat that's found deep in your abdominal region where it can wrap around your stomach, liver, and intestines, and negatively influence how these and other nearby organs work. Visceral fat is considered a harmful and "active" fat because it releases inflammatory proteins that may ultimately lead to a chronic low-grade level of inflammation.

When visceral fat cells release damaging and destructive proteins into the body, the result can be inflamed tissues, narrowed blood vessels, higher levels of LDL cholesterol, and insulin resistance. These factors are linked to increased risk of developing atherosclerosis (arterial plaque), cognitive impairment, cardiovascular disease, and type 2 diabetes.

The problem is that as we age, and especially as we approach and enter menopause, we become much more susceptible to gaining visceral fat. Researchers haven't determined why exactly this happens, but it seems to be a result of a combination of factors including normal aging, changes in diet and level of activity, decline in sleep quality, and—since it is a key regulator of fat—diminished estrogen. As our estrogen levels wane during the menopausal transition, a shift in the type of fat we gain takes place and we are more likely to put on pounds made up of visceral fat. One study determined that a premenopausal woman's total body fat is likely to be 5 to 8 percent visceral fat, whereas a postmenopausal woman's total body fat is 15 to 20 percent visceral fat. Given the links between visceral fat and disease, this is a percentage that should get our attention and inspire us to act; in the Tool Kit, I'll show you some of the most effective strategies I've found to combat visceral fat gain.

KNOW YOUR RISKS

You can gain visceral fat over your lifetime as a result of excess calorie intake (relative to less activity), routine sedentary behavior, and exposure to prolonged stress that increases production of cortisol, a stress hormone that can promote abdominal obesity. And it's obvious too that in midlife, decreased estrogen can play a big role in setting us up to store fat deep in the belly region.

KNOW YOUR NUMBERS

Visceral fat doesn't reveal itself in numbers on the scale, which is why it can be tough to measure. But to be completely honest with you, I'm okay with not using a scale to determine where I stand, and I don't recommend it to my patients either. I think we have spent way too much time focusing on numbers on a scale or fighting against fat gain—at least I know that's all I used to pay attention to, and I've had to work hard to train my brain away from the scale as a measure of progress (I now prefer to focus on how much muscle I have—see next point on why this is the case).

The easiest and most inexpensive way to get an approximation of visceral fat is to calculate your waist-to-hip ratio. This isn't going to give you a precise visceral fat percentage, but it can help give you a sense of how your body might be changing in response to shifting hormone levels. To get your waist-to-hip ratio, first get a tape measure and then:

- Get your waist circumference by measuring the distance around the smallest part of your waist. This is usually just above your belly button.

- Get your hip circumference by measuring the largest part of your hips.

- Calculate your waist-to-hip ratio by dividing your waist circumference by your hip circumference.

- Use this chart to help you determine if you may have a measurement of abdominal obesity that may put you at increased health risk:

HEALTH RISK	WAIST-TO-HIP RATIO (WOMEN)
Low	0.80 or lower
Moderate	0.81-0.85
High	0.86 or higher

You may also be able to seek out a clinic or specialized provider who offers a type of scan that measures your body composition. This may be the DEXA scan, which can look at bone density, visceral fat, and muscle mass, or the similar InBody Scan (see more on these in the next section).

HOW MHT MAY HELP

The research on hormone therapy and its effect on abdominal obesity has produced some positive results. It's been shown to be effective in reducing levels of visceral fat and in helping prevent age-related weight gain in early postmenopausal women. The caveat is that when MHT is stopped, the positive impact on weight gain seems to disappear, making other strategies essential.

Sarcopenia

The other body composition change that occurs during the menopausal transition, often in tandem with visceral fat gain, is the progressive loss of lean mass or muscle tissue, a condition that eventually leads to sarcopenia. Sarcopenia is a progressive age-related condition characterized by the loss of skeletal muscle mass, strength, and function. It often contributes to reduced physical performance and an increased risk of falls and fractures, affecting overall quality of life.

As you approach or pass menopause, your muscle tissue can begin to lose quality and strength, a process that's driven by increasing inflammation (in part due to gains in visceral fat), aging, insulin resistance, and the loss of estrogen. Estrogen plays an important role in muscle tissue maintenance that is similar to its role in bone remodeling: It helps muscle tissue regenerate and rebuild. So when estrogen levels decline in menopause, your muscle tissue mass begins to decline as well. Muscle loss can lead to decreased mobility and strength, increased fat mass, and generally poorer metabolic health. Losing muscle can also increase the risk of falls and fractures as you age.

KNOW YOUR RISKS

Clinical sarcopenia is most commonly diagnosed in individuals sixty-five and older, but muscle loss begins to happen much earlier, around the age of thirty. After thirty, it's estimated that we lose between 3 and 5 percent of our muscle mass each decade, and this accelerates to up to 10 percent after menopause. Your risk for sarcopenia goes up after menopause, and additional risk factors include type 2 diabetes, smoking, physical inactivity, and malnutrition.

KNOW YOUR NUMBERS

There's currently no good screening test for sarcopenia, and unfortunately it doesn't get diagnosed until it's fairly advanced. If your doctor suspects you are at risk for sarcopenia, they might run tests to check your grip strength and calf circumference and ultimately order a CT scan to look at your muscle mass.

You may also be able to seek out a clinic or specialized provider who offers a type of scan that measures your body composition. This may be the DEXA scan, which can look at bone density, visceral fat, and muscle mass. In my clinic, we rely on a similar tool called the InBody Scan to help determine a patient's muscle mass and risk of sarcopenia.

Ultimately, I don't think anyone should wait to get a test that confirms the presence or risk of sarcopenia—it's better to understand that muscle loss is inevitable with age and the sooner we take steps to build and maintain muscle, the better.

HOW MHT MAY HELP

MHT has been found to have significant positive effects on muscle mass and strength. Specifically, hormone therapy has shown to increase estrogen receptors in the muscle and help improve muscle power, contraction, and composition. These benefits are most pronounced in women who start MHT closer to menopause. We will discuss other strategies to combat muscle mass/strength loss during menopause (and before) in the Tool Kit.

The Health Risks We Can't Ignore

Everything you experience during menopause starts with the decline of ovarian function and the resulting reduction in estrogen production (and some other key hormones too, but estrogen has by far the most impact). The loss of estrogen can lead to a long list of noticeable symptoms, and it's important that we find ways to feel better. As we pay attention to symptoms, however, I want to make sure that we don't lose sight of the under-the-radar changes that are also taking place and may be shifting our internal systems toward dysfunction and disease. In menopause, we must prioritize the prevention of osteoporosis, coronary artery disease, insulin resistance and prediabetes, neuroinflammation, visceral fat gain, and sarcopenia (loss of muscle mass). Our longevity depends upon it!

CHAPTER 7

Everything You Wanted to Know About Hormone Therapy

Menopause at forty? Was that even possible for me? I was getting my period every twenty-one days for about five months, and then: nothing! I took a pregnancy test, negative. Then the hot flashes started like a raging fire. At night I changed my pajamas and bed sheets while my husband slept, oblivious of the anguish I was going through. My GP advised me to return in a year, and she would consider HRT. She said to me, "Well you are a runner, so hopefully your bones will be strong." I was stunned—that's all you have to say? Was this the beginning of osteoporosis and cardiovascular risks, and brain and mental health concerns? My doctor gave no more details about how this would be a serious roller-coaster ride. For a year, I suffered needlessly with hot flashes, brain fog, low libido, anxiety and panic attacks. What in the world was happening to me? She prescribed HRT until "you reach the natural age of menopause, which is fifty." But once I was on HRT, I felt so good on HRT! Thankfully another provider prescribed HRT. I'm fifty-four and still taking it.

—Sue D.

All right, it's time to roll up our sleeves and get into the details on hormone therapy. This is a *big* subject, so I'll focus on the areas where I get the most questions, including the different types of MHT, options for delivering them to your body, when to begin and/or end usage, and who is a good candidate for their use.

My goal with this chapter is to establish a foundation of information that allows you to better understand your options when it comes to hormone replacement therapy, and to advocate for yourself as you seek support from your own healthcare provider. I think that to achieve this goal we must first take a step back and go over some hormone basics.

A Note to Healthcare Professionals

I know that there may be healthcare professionals reading this chapter because you were never taught how to prescribe hormone replacement therapy and want to learn how to do it. Or maybe you just want to become more informed on the topic because your patients are asking for guidance. I hope the information in this chapter is helpful but want to caution that this content is not intended to deliver clinical guidelines and/or inform how you practice medicine. However, I absolutely encourage you to check out the Menopause Society's certification program. If you are a licensed healthcare practitioner, such as a physician, physician assistant, nurse practitioner, nurse, pharmacist, or psychologist, you can complete the program to become a Certified Menopause Practitioner (CMP).

If you promote menopause care as a part of your practice, but you are not planning on seeking certification from the Menopause Society, or screening for perimenopause/menopause and offering treatment options (and those options should NOT be limited to pellet therapy), you should consider removing menopause care from your scope of practice.

Hormones 101

Hormones are chemical messengers that tell your cells what to do. Your cells have internal or surface-based receptors, which allow them to receive communication from your hormones and to follow the instructions as delivered. The instructions may be to metabolize fuel, rebuild tissue, or perform other tasks that are vital to keeping the machine that is your body in top form. When hormone levels decline because of disease, age, or the menopausal transition, cells and tissues can be left waiting to be told what to do, and essential tasks may not get completed—this is when trouble can start.

Where Hormones Come From

Your body relies on several systems to keep it up and running. One of these systems is called the endocrine system, which is made up of the pituitary gland, pineal gland, hypothalamus gland, thyroid gland, adrenal glands, pancreas, testes, and ovaries. This is your hormone specialty team, and it's responsible for the production and release of dozens of hormones that influence almost every cell and function in the body. During your menopausal transition, your ovaries and the hypothalamus and pituitary glands undergo the most change.

What Hormones Are Most Relevant in Menopause?

During menopause, your body naturally reduces production of three main hormone groups: estrogens, progesterone, and androgens. Let's learn a little more about this important trio. (Don't worry—there will not be a quiz at the end of this chapter! I just want to make sure you are familiar with the terms that may come up as you research hormone therapy.)

ESTROGENS

We tend to talk about estrogen as though it is a single hormone, but there are actually three major estrogens produced in the body: estradiol, estrone, and estriol. Each of these has a distinct impact on certain functions throughout the body.

Estradiol is the primary estrogen secreted by the ovaries during the reproductive or premenopausal phase of life, and its production almost completely disappears after menopause. It's the most biologically active and strongest of the estrogens, meaning it has the biggest impact within the body. In most cases, when people are talking about estrogen, they are referring to estradiol.

Estriol is produced by a developing placenta during pregnancy and is mostly undetectable in nonpregnant individuals. Still, even at low levels, it can affect bone health and lipid management.

Estrone is considered the weakest of the estrogens and is produced mostly in small amounts by the ovaries. When the ovaries start to produce less estrone during menopause, your body has a work-around: The adrenal glands release more of a substance that your fat tissue can convert into estrone. Thanks to this creative alternative method of production, estrone becomes the most prominent form of natural estrogen in the body after menopause. In postmenopause, estrone may help slightly reduce bone loss and aid in tissue maintenance, but unfortunately it won't be able to step in and do the complete job of estradiol.

PROGESTERONE

Progesterone is the hormone produced by the ovary after ovulation and by the placenta during pregnancy. Its most important job during our reproductive years is to prepare the uterus to support and sustain a pregnancy. It also has important functions in maintaining our moods and sleep optimization. Loss of progesterone after menopause is linked to increased levels of depression, anxiety, and insomnia.

In the context of hormone therapy, the word you'll likely hear used is *progestogens*. This category includes both bioidentical progesterone and progestins, which are the synthetic versions made to emulate the properties of naturally occurring progesterone; they get close, but they aren't identical to what's made in the body.

ANDROGENS

Androgens are hormones produced mostly by the ovaries and the adrenal gland (with a little also made within fat and other tissues). The most significant of these are testosterone, androstenedione, and dehydroepiandrosterone (DHEA). While androgens are most typically associated with development in men and male characteristics, they play a critical role for everyone in the areas of energy, mood, libido, and muscle tone and mass. As we approach and reach ovarian failure during menopause, we experience a decrease in androgen levels, which can lead to depressive feelings, decreased sex drive, and increased fatigue. Androgen production tapers off during menopause, but it doesn't drop off entirely. It can even continue to be produced in postmenopause—that is, unless you need to have a bilateral oophorectomy (the removal of both ovaries). That surgery will lead to a rapid decline in testosterone levels, which may result in more severe symptoms, despite your still getting DHEA and androstenedione from the adrenal gland. The profound loss of testosterone is one of the reasons I always advise very careful consideration of hormone therapy if you are faced with the potential need to have both ovaries removed.

Defining Hormone Replacement Therapy

You may have noticed that hormone therapy goes by a lot of names. Some experts use the term *hormone therapy* (HT), and it used to be referred to as *hormone replacement therapy* (HRT). I prefer to use *menopausal hormone therapy* (MHT) as a broad term to describe the use of hormone replacement during perimenopause and postmenopause.

The Benefit-Versus-Risk Ratio

The most important consideration for menopausal hormone therapy (MHT) use is each person's benefit-versus-risk ratio; in the ideal candidate for hormone therapy, the benefits will outweigh the risks. Since estrogen replacement specifically delivers the greatest benefits to menopausal individuals, the question of risk should be focused there. Ideally, your doctor will consider you as an individual and ask: What are the risks of estrogen use for my patient? And what are the strategies for risk reduction? If you have a uterus, you should never ever receive estrogen alone because of the risk of endometrial hyperplasia/cancer from unopposed estrogen. The absolute standard for reducing this risk is taking a progestogen along with estrogen. If your doctor does not support this combined therapy, find another doctor immediately.

I will get more into this and how you can determine if you're a candidate for MHT starting on page 105.

When to Consider "Replacing" Your Hormones

If you are symptomatic, you can begin hormone replacement therapy anywhere in your menopausal journey, and the earlier the better. Yes, this means that you can begin using hormone therapy in perimenopause, and you can experience the benefits of MHT *before your periods stop.* During perimenopause, fluctuating levels of estrogen and progesterone can often lead to hot flashes, night sweats, mood swings, and irregular menstrual cycles, and hormone therapy is highly effective at reducing these symptoms and improving quality of life. This is why for my patients, I recommend MHT—as long as the benefits outweigh the risks for the individual—as soon as any symptoms present and that includes perimenopause.

But what if you don't have symptoms and feel fine? It's possible that you too should consider it because of the potential health benefits (protecting your brain, heart, bones, vagina, and bladder, as well as lowering your risk of death from any cause). Again, timing is critical: For some women starting late will not confer any benefits on the heart or brain and may make existing diseases in those organs worse (we discussed the timing/healthy cell hypothesis earlier in chapter 3).

There is currently no set recommended age or duration at which you should stop using hormone therapy—but again, the question of risks versus benefits should be asked ideally at every healthcare visit beginning in perimenopause. Whether we like it or not, we are all aging, and this active process can bring about changes in our bodies that require us to revisit what may be the best and safest strategies for minimizing the symptoms and health risks of menopause.

The Difference Between a Birth Control Pill and MHT

The birth control pill (often referred to as "combined birth control") and menopause hormone therapies are both made up of the same basic hormones—estrogens and progestogens—which is why many patients come in asking me if they can't just continue taking the pill. The primary difference in these medications is *dosage*. MHT was developed to control the symptoms of menopause, and birth control pills were developed to suppress ovulation and prevent pregnancy; you need much higher doses to accomplish the latter. When I see people on social media demonizing hormonal contraception as "dangerous" when they are the first to encourage menopausal hormone therapy, I have to wonder if they truly understand the difference.

For some in perimenopause, the ovulation-suppressing dosage in a birth control pill may be the preferred approach to symptom relief. For example, if I have a patient suffering from menorrhagia, or heavy irregular cycles, I will often want to suppress her ovulations with the doses found in hormonal birth control if other causes of menorrhagia have been ruled out. There are also progestin-only forms (no estrogen) of contraception, which in special cases may be used during perimenopause to alleviate symptoms.

What this means is that if you are experiencing perimenopausal symptoms, you have options that can be customized to your distinct health history, symptoms, and preferences. If you don't have access to an informed healthcare provider, keep looking—they are out there! You can also visit my website at thepauselife.com to find a growing list of providers in your area.

Types of Hormone Therapy

Synthetic Versus Bioidentical

There are a lot of terms tossed around in the hormone therapy space and this can make it very confusing. You might hear *conventional, traditional, natural, unnatural* . . . the list goes on and on. I think the easiest way to categorize types of MHT is to understand them as your body does: as either synthetic or bioidentical.

Synthetic hormones are made from chemical compounds. They do not have the same molecular structure as the original sex hormones in your body, so your body converts them into usable form.

Bioidentical hormones are made from naturally derived ingredients and are usually plant derived. They are structurally identical to those naturally produced by the body.

Both synthetic and bioidentical hormones are made in a lab, but I prefer bioidentical formulations for my patients, as it makes sense to me to "give them back the water they were drinking." When we are talking about MHT, the bioidentical hormones on the "menu" are versions of estradiol, progesterone, and testosterone.

Now, within the bioidentical hormone therapy (BHT or BHRT) space, there are two categories: compounded bioidentical hormone therapy and FDA-approved bioidentical hormone therapy. It's important to understand how they differ.

Compounded Bioidentical Versus FDA-Approved Bioidentical

The hormones of *compounded bioidentical hormone therapy* are mixed and prepared in a compounding pharmacy. This type of hormone therapy is considered to be customized to the individual since it allows for healthcare providers to adjust the hormone dosage and delivery system (e.g., cream, gel, capsule, troche).

The catch is that compounding pharmacies are not subject to the same rigorous regulatory oversight as pharmaceutical manufacturers. Quality control may vary from one compounding pharmacy to another, and there have been instances of inconsistent dosages or contamination. This raises concerns about the safety, purity, and consistency of compounded hormone preparations, so the FDA does not approve these prescriptions. As a result, compounded hormones are typically not covered by insurance and must be paid for out of pocket.

The hormones of *FDA-approved bioidentical hormone therapy* are commercially manufactured by pharmaceutical companies following strict regulatory guidelines. They are manufactured as standardized medications with precise dosages and forms (meaning they do not allow for customization). This type of hormone therapy is offered only by prescription and is typically covered by insurance. FDA-approved hormone products also undergo rigorous testing (often involving trials with large groups of patients) and are known to be consistent in terms of dosing and quality.

I think the fact that compounding pharmacies offer customization is fantastic, and I will prescribe compounded therapy if FDA-regulated options haven't worked for my patients (which may be the case if they have an allergy or need a customized dose). However, I suggest being wary of any claims that promote compounded hormones as better or safer than noncompounded varieties. In the past, the FDA has had to issue warning letters to a number of compounding pharmacies about making false, unsupported claims, specifically their claim that compounded bioidentical hormone therapy options containing estriol, such as BiEST and TriEST, are safer than FDA-approved options made with other estrogens. These products contain 20 percent estradiol and 80 percent estriol, and because estriol is a weaker estrogen, the promise is that this ratio is safer for tissues in the breast and/or uterus. I'm all for reduced risk, but unfortunately this claim has not been supported by clinical trials, and the reality is that estriol still has a stimulatory effect on the breast and endometrium.

The other thing about compounding pharmacies is that they present a sales opportunity for promoters of unreliable hormone testing practices. There are practitioners out there who will promote the use of saliva- or urine-based testing, namely the DUTCH urine test (which costs hundreds of out-of-pocket dollars), to help them promote customized prescriptions for hormone therapy—and these practitioners rely exclusively on compounding pharmacies. Yet the hormone tests they're using aren't accurate or effective as a means of determining the most effective dosing for a patient. This is because your hormone levels change day to day and can vary wildly during the menopausal transition—there's simply no way to pin the right dose on the moving target that is your hormones during this time of your life. The smarter strategy is to start with the lowest possible dose of any FDA-approved medication and wait three to four weeks to see if symptoms improve. If they don't, that's when adjustments in dose and/or medication are made.

Hormone Therapy Delivery Systems

We've covered the hormones that go into menopause hormone therapies, as well as the options for their manufacture. Another key factor to consider is what *delivery system* to use. In an ideal world, your doctor will discuss delivery system options with you and advise on the best type of therapy for you. However, since so many women have shared with me directly that they are not even being granted the discussion of MHT, I can be 100 percent certain that they are not getting an explanation of all the options that exist. So I'm going to offer maybe more detail here than is necessary because I want you to know what's available and what questions you can ask so you can become a better advocate for yourself.

Estrogens

There are two ways estrogen replacement therapy can be delivered to the body: systemically and locally (vaginally).

SYSTEMIC MEDICATIONS

Systemic medications go into the bloodstream through a pill or cream or gel or patch and affect all body tissues. Since they have an overall effect, they can deliver greater relief, but this can come with increased risk of side effects. Systemic options come in many different delivery forms.

There is one *oral* option:

- PILL: the most convenient form, yet because of an effect on the liver (see sidebar on page 97), this creates a slightly increased risk of clotting, hypertension, and abnormal triglycerides.

There are multiple *nonoral* options, some FDA approved and some not. The FDA-approved options are:

- PATCH: applied to the skin with an adhesive

- GEL: rubbed into skin daily

- RING: inserted into vagina and worn continuously for three months

- SPRAY: applied to skin daily

- INJECTION: The estradiol cypionate and estradiol valerate forms of long-acting estrogen injection come as a liquid to inject into a muscle. These medications are usually injected by a healthcare professional once every three to four weeks. I don't use these in my practice because of cost to the patient and inconvenience.

The non-FDA-approved options are:

- CREAM: compounded, rubbed into skin daily

- PELLETS: preloaded with testosterone plus or minus estrogens and injected under the skin, replaced every three to four months. See the sidebar on page 102 for more about pellets.

- TROCHES: A troche is like a lozenge. It's designed to be placed between your cheek and your gums, where the skin lining is very thin. In this position it gradually dissolves, releasing its active ingredients directly into your circulatory system.

The Risks of Oral Estrogen

When you take medication orally (by mouth), it goes through your digestive system before entering your bloodstream. In the case of oral estrogen, the medication is processed by the liver before reaching the rest of the body. This initial processing in the liver is called the "first-pass effect." There are well-established risks associated with this oral estrogen and the liver-first route of processing, including

- *Hypertension (high blood pressure):* Oral estrogen can lead to higher levels of certain proteins in the blood, which may interrupt normal blood vessel function and contribute to elevated blood pressure.

- *Increased risk of clotting:* When estrogen is processed in the liver, it can create a procoagulant state in your bloodstream by increasing the production of substances that promote blood clot formation. Then, if blood clots form excessively, it can lead to an increased risk of conditions like deep vein thrombosis (blood clots in the legs) or pulmonary embolism (blood clots in the lungs), or thrombotic strokes.

It's extremely important that your doctor evaluate your personal risk factors when considering the route of hormone replacement therapy that's right for you. I generally don't recommend oral estrogen because of the risks mentioned, and I especially don't prescribe it if a patient has a personal or genetic history of clotting disorders or high blood pressure (even if it's controlled through the use of medication). Instead, I like to prescribe nonoral forms of estrogen, such as skin patches, gels, or vaginal rings, which are proven to be safer because they bypass the liver during their initial journey into the bloodstream.

LOCAL MEDICATIONS

Local medications are topical and inserted into the vagina. Local forms of MHT are low dose, typically have low to no risks, and are used to directly treat vaginal and/or urinary symptoms of menopause. You absolutely can use vaginal estrogen *with* systemic estrogen; in fact, many of my patients do! I recommend vaginal estrogen as first-line therapy to all patients who have any signs of vaginal atrophy. Your options for local medications may include:

- CREAM: inserted into the vagina at least once a week. Most women tolerate this well, but for some the alcohol base may cause irritation.

- TABLET: inserted into vagina at least once a week.

- RING: inserted into vagina every three months. I love this one because it is so convenient and well tolerated, but it's rarely covered by insurance.

- SUPPOSITORY: FDA approved, inserted into vagina at least once a week.

All of these options come in both FDA-approved and compound pharmacy forms.

SERMs: "Designer" Estrogens

If you've had breast cancer or are at increased risk for estrogen receptor–positive breast cancer (ERPB) and are seeking relief for menopausal symptoms, your doctor may recommend to you a "SERM" such as tamoxifen or raloxifene. *SERM* stands for *selective estrogen receptor modulator*, and these medications work by blocking the effects of estrogen in certain tissues and providing the benefits of estrogen in others. For example, they can block estrogen's effect on breast tissue, as in the case of some breast cancer treatments, without increasing the risk of other tissues like bone or endometrium.

SERMs may also be used if you:

- are at risk of osteoporosis but cannot take estrogen. Likely medication: raloxifene

- have a history of blood clots or are at higher risk for cardiovascular events. Likely medication: raloxifene

- are experiencing vaginal symptoms, such as dryness, itching, or painful intercourse, and topical estrogen isn't a desired option. Likely medication: oral ospemifene (Osphena)

- have a personal preference or a contraindication for MHT (see list on page 108). Likely medication: Duavee, a SERM that combines estrogen with bazedoxifene to protect the uterus. For patients who cannot tolerate progestogens, this can be a good option, as it also protects the lining of the uterus and negates the need for a progestogen.

Progestogens

Progesterone plays a crucial role in hormone therapy during perimeno-pause and menopause, and if you still have your uterus, it is essential to use it in combination with estrogen replacement therapy. Estrogen has a thick-ening effect on the uterine lining, which can become abnormal if it's allowed to continue unopposed. Progesterone is introduced to directly oppose estrogen's effects on the endometrium, which helps counteract the risk. Progesterone can also help alleviate hot flashes, headaches, night sweats, mood swings, and vaginal dryness. As I mentioned earlier, progestogens include both bioidentical progesterone and the synthetic progestins.

There are a couple ways that progesterone may be prescribed. There's what's referred to as sequential therapy, which is when you take a progestogen for a specific time frame (e.g., ten to fourteen days each month) to mimic the natural progesterone surge that occurs after ovulation. I don't use this in practice because I find it's too confusing and can lead to disrupted dosing. I recommend continuous therapy, which is when you take a progestogen daily. Progestogens can also be incredibly helpful for sleep, even if not "required" because of lack of a uterus or the presence of a progestin-containing IUD. The options for therapy (progesterone spray, suppository, oral forms, and troches) can all be compounded.

Oral forms (pills) include:

- ORAL MICRONIZED PROGESTERONE: bioidentical formulation.

- SYNTHETIC PROGESTINS: usually combined with an estrogen for either MHT or combined oral contraception. Progestin-only oral contraceptive options are available as well.

Nonoral forms include:

- TRANSDERMAL CREAM: cream offered only by compounding pharmacies.

- PATCH: FDA approved, usually formulated as a synthetic progestin with an estrogen for menopausal hormone therapy, or in a combined contraceptive patch.

- INJECTIONS: non-FDA approved, progesterone in oil.

- VAGINAL GEL: FDA approved, usually used for fertility purposes.

- PROGESTIN-CONTAINING IUDS: progestin-containing intrauterine devices that release a progestin directly into the uterus, reducing the risk of endometrial abnormalities. Not for systemic therapy, only for local therapy.

Transdermal Progesterone: Not Enough Protection

Transdermal bioidentical progesterone is a cream-based compounded progesterone that you apply to your skin. It is a popular option with certain practitioners, but I don't prescribe it because this form of progesterone does not offer adequate protection against endometrial hyperplasia and cancer when combined with estrogen replacement therapy. This is because the progesterone molecule is quite large and is poorly absorbed through the skin, and research has shown that not enough of it makes it into your body to help counter the effect of estrogen therapy on the uterus, putting you at increased risk of endometrial hyperplasia and cancer.

Androgens

TESTOSTERONE

In an ideal world, there would be an FDA-approved testosterone option for women that doses this hormone in female-appropriate amounts, that's available, is easy to prescribe, and is covered by insurance, but . . . well, that ideal world doesn't exist just yet. Given that testosterone has been shown to improve sexual functioning, muscle tone and mass, fatigue, and bone health in menopausal women, we can hope that one day there will be an FDA-approved version. Until then, many practitioners, myself included, are prescribing the off-label use of testosterone for some of our menopausal patients.

For many of my patients, a compounded testosterone cream has proven to be the best option. Other doctors may recommend pellets inserted subcutaneously (see sidebar below), or sublingual (under the tongue) and buccal (between the teeth and gums) formulations in the form of troches.

It's critical that no matter how you deliver testosterone to your body, if you decide to do so, you be routinely monitored for adverse events and make sure you avoid dosing that supersedes what may naturally be found in the body.

Most forms of oral testosterone are not FDA approved and should not be used due to potential for severe liver toxicity. Testosterone undecanoate is a safer oral option that has been studied in menopausal women for hypoactive sexual desire disorder, and did show improvement.

Nonoral forms include:

- INJECTIONS: FDA approved for men under limited medical circumstances but not for women

- PATCH: FDA approved for men, no lower dose available for women

- GEL: FDA approved for men, may be given in lower doses for women

- CREAMS: not FDA approved; compounded, usually applied to thighs once a day

- PELLETS: compounded only (see below)

What's the Deal with Biote Pellets?

There's a popular form of testosterone therapy on the market called Biote. Biote is pellet based and requires a small incision to be made in your gluteal area where the pellets may be inserted. I know people find this approach appealing because it doesn't require regular application of a cream, but there are a number of risks and side effects to consider.

The primary risk of testosterone pellets is related to the fact that they can administer what's referred to as a supraphysiological dose and can lead to a much higher than normal level of testosterone that is naturally found in females. In fact, the makers of Biote target total serum testosterone levels of 150–250 nanograms per deciliter (ng/dL) for females when normal healthy levels are between 15–70 ng/dL. I have seen patients in my clinic who have lingering testosterone levels above 300 ng/dL (well into the male range of 260–1000 ng/dL) months after pellet insertion. There just haven't been well-controlled studies or evidence to support testosterone levels this high in females. And higher-than-normal dosing of testosterone in women can lead to:

- increased body hair growth, deepening of the voice, and an enlargement of the clitoris

- acne and oily skin

- mood swings, irritability, and aggression

- an increase in LDL cholesterol (the "bad" cholesterol) and a decrease in HDL cholesterol (the "good" cholesterol), a combination that increases the risk of heart disease

- liver damage and/or liver tumors, fatty liver, and elevated liver enzymes

- irregular periods or halted menstruation

- increased risk of blood clots

- increasing levels of visceral fat

Your doctor may safely prescribe a physiologic dose (a dose of medication that brings you to the range of a normal healthy woman) of testosterone to bring diminished levels back up to "normal," which is likely to have a lesser degree of risk. You could be prescribed testosterone for hypoactive sexual desire disorder (HSDD) or sexual dysfunction, or off label for fatigue, osteoporosis, or sarcopenia. The challenge is that testosterone therapy is still relatively new in women, and we don't really have a solid grasp on what "normal" levels are for women in their menopausal journey and how supplementation will be tolerated long term. If a discussion with your doctor leads to you choosing supplemental testosterone, be sure that part of your follow-up includes regular blood work to check your testosterone levels.

DHEA

DHEA (dehydroepiandrosterone) is a steroid hormone produced by the adrenal glands and in smaller amounts by the ovaries. DHEA acts as a precursor to estradiol, initially converting into androstenedione, which is further metabolized into testosterone and estradiol through enzymatic processes within the body. There has been growing interest in the use of supplemental DHEA to help relieve menopausal symptoms (I definitely get a lot of questions on the topic!).

There have been studies showing that intravaginal DHEA supplementation can help a great deal in relieving vaginal pain or discomfort in menopause. It's also proven to help relieve hot flashes and night sweats, support immune function, and increase muscle mass, and it may potentially help reduce bone loss. However, the jury is still out as to whether it has any benefits in the areas of cardiovascular disease, insulin sensitivity, cognitive function, or adrenal insufficiency.

We have also yet to see evidence that DHEA can increase testosterone levels. For this reason, I currently do not recommend oral DHEA supplementation to my patients to boost their testosterone levels. If we decide to therapeutically increase a patient's testosterone levels, I prescribe testosterone.

The *oral form* (pills) of DHEA is not FDA approved and is sold over the counter as a supplement.

DHEA is also sold in *nonoral form* as a vaginal suppository. Intrarosa (prasterone) is FDA approved for moderate to severe pain during sexual intercourse, a symptom of vulvar and vaginal atrophy.

A Word on DIM

Diindolylmethane (DIM) is a compound found in cruciferous vegetables such as broccoli, cauliflower, and Brussels sprouts. There's been increasing interest, especially in the integrative medicine space, in the use of concentrated doses of DIM in supplement form to help "balance" hormones and potentially relieve symptoms of menopause. I have yet to see conclusive evidence to support its use, which is why I don't recommend it to my patients. And I advise others to approach with caution bold claims on the ability of DIM to resolve hormone issues or prevent cancer—we simply don't know enough about it yet.

I think it's tempting to take something that might have benefits (even though they're not scientifically proven), but it's important to note there can be unknown side effects and risks involved. In some individuals, DIM supplements may lead to gastrointestinal discomfort, headaches, or allergic reaction, and they can interfere with certain medications, especially those metabolized by the liver. Until we have stronger science to support the use of DIM in supplement form, I recommend that you get your daily dose of diindolylmethane from cruciferous vegetables themselves—they're safer and definitely more delicious.

Getting Started with MHT: Formulations and Dosing

It's the job of your doctor or prescribing provider to help identify the best formulations for you, but I want to make one thing very clear: There are numerous FDA-approved options available to you as a patient. If you are being offered only one option, you need to ask why and consider if sales of this option might be benefiting your healthcare practitioner in some way. If you get any kind of indirect or evasive answer, consider finding another doctor.

Resources for MHT Formulations on the Market

The pharmaceutical formulations of MHT are abundant and they are constantly being updated, so it's impossible to give you a current list in print form. Instead, I suggest you check out the following resources for the most current and comprehensive list of options:

From the Menopause Society (TMS), for patients (free): https://www.menopause.org/docs/default-source/professional/menonote-deciding-about-ht-2022.pdf

From TMS, for patients and providers (requires payment to access): https://www.menopause.org/publications/professional-publications/em -menopause-practice-em-textbook

From the FDA, for patients and providers (free): https://www.fda.gov /consumers/free-publications-women/menopause-medicines-help-you

---

In my practice, I discuss the possible formulations with each of my patients (and I of course base the prescription specifics on individual intake forms and relevant testing), but I also have established "go-to" formulations. These are selected on the basis of cost to the patient, convenience, and safety. They include:

- ESTRADIOL PATCH: typically covered by insurance, out of pocket with various coupons. Averages about $30/month.

- ORAL MICRONIZED PROGESTERONE (in patients with intact uterus): typically covered by insurance, out of pocket with various coupons. Averages about $10/month, more if nonstandard dosing is needed.

- COMPOUNDED TESTOSTERONE CREAM: never covered by insurance. Averages about $30/month.

When it comes to MHT, dosing can make all the difference; too little can be ineffective, and too much can increase the risk of unwanted side effects. Unfortunately, there's no universal starting point when it comes to the ideal dose, but some guidelines have been established based on patient type.

Generally, symptomatic patients who are ten or fewer years removed from menopause often do better at higher doses. And patients who are more than ten years removed from menopause can benefit from starting with lower doses. This latter group may do well on a lower dose because (hopefully) their symptoms are less severe than what may be experienced in early menopause. Lower doses can also minimize potential risks, which increase the further away you are from menopause. When my patients have significant risk factors for potential coronary artery disease, for example, if they are ten or more years removed from menopause or over the age of sixty, I recommend a coronary calcium score test prior to beginning therapy.

The Frustrating Facts on MHT Costs

There are shocking discrepancies when it comes to the costs of medications in this country, and menopausal hormone therapy is no exception. It's a frustrating reality, but if you want the best price, you're going to have to put in some hustle and legwork. I have to compare and chase down decent prices for my own meds: I get Celebrex (an anti-inflammatory) from a local grocery store with a coupon from Good Rx, which allows me to save hundreds a year. My MHT is shipped to me from a mail-order pharmacy using my insurance, and I pay out of pocket for my testosterone at a local compounding pharmacy after cost comparison.

I wish that we could just pick up all we needed from our local pharmacy using insurance and all pay the same reasonable costs, but the system is truly broken (except for when it comes to generic Viagra, which you can get for pennies a day wherever you get it!).

My best advice is to go into sorting out the specifics of your MHT protocol with an open mind. Since there is no one-size-fits-all approach, achieving what's right for you will require a trial-and-error process, and that demands patience—this can be a lot to ask if you've been symptomatic for some time and you are desperate for relief. The right dose for you does exist; it just might take time to land there. An informed menopause practitioner will help dial in your dosing on the basis of how your symptoms respond, that is, how you feel, so you'll want to keep tabs on any noticeable side effects or improvements as you begin using MHT or your dosing is adjusted.

Who Should Not Use MHT

Since 2002 there has been a stubborn narrative in place that MHT is dangerous to your health, specifically that it puts you at high risk of developing breast cancer and heart disease. This inaccurate idea, planted in people's minds courtesy of the reporting surrounding the Women's Health Initiative (WHI) study, has turned countless women away from the relief and improved quality of life that can be gained through the use of hormone therapy. What's come to light since then is that for most menopausal women who are less than ten years out from menopause, MHT is not only safe but also the single most effective way to minimize symptoms and reduce the health risks that come with the hormone changes that occur during the menopausal transition. (For all the details of the WHI study, revisit chapter 3.)

Now, "most" women does not mean all women. There are absolute contraindications when it comes to hormone therapy use. A contraindication is a specific condition or reason that a drug or procedure should not be used because it may be harmful to the person. You should not use MHT if the following safety concerns are present:

- KNOWN OR SUSPECTED BREAST CANCER OR OTHER ESTROGEN- OR PROGESTOGEN-SENSITIVE CANCER: MHT can stimulate the growth of hormone-sensitive cancers, so it's not recommended for individuals with a history of these types of cancers.

- UNDIAGNOSED ABNORMAL GENITAL BLEEDING: Any unexplained unusual vaginal bleeding needs proper diagnosis before considering MHT, as it could be a sign of an underlying condition.

- ACTIVE OR RECENT ARTERIAL THROMBOEMBOLIC DISEASE: Conditions like recent heart attack or stroke pose risks when combined with oral MHT, as it may further increase the risk of blood clots.

- ACTIVE OR RECENT VENOUS THROMBOEMBOLIC DISEASE: Conditions like deep vein thrombosis or pulmonary embolism can be aggravated by oral hormone therapy, leading to further clotting risks.

- KNOWN OR SUSPECTED PREGNANCY: Hormone therapy is not appropriate during pregnancy because of potential effects on fetal development.

- ACTIVE SEVERE LIVER DISEASE OR DYSFUNCTION: Individuals with significant liver impairment might not metabolize hormones properly, making MHT unsafe.

- HYPERSENSITIVITY TO ANY COMPONENTS OF HORMONE THERAPY: Prior allergic reactions to components of MHT can prohibit you from using them again.

MHT should not be used if any of these specific conditions are met because the risks for the patient are known to be greater than the benefits.

It's important to note that the same exclusion does not extend to related conditions. I point this out because there are plenty of reports (including thousands of comments on my social media posts) of well-meaning healthcare providers who have stretched this list of contraindications and excluded patients from MHT because of a sort of guilt-by-association logic. Some of the most common misconceptions are the following:

1. **A history of endometriosis automatically excludes you from MHT.** FALSE. The treatment of menopause (surgical or natural) with a history of endometriosis remains controversial. A 2023 review suggests that there is risk of endometriosis recurrence in estrogen-only HRT in patients who had pelvic clearance (TAH/BSO) as disease treatment. A patient with a history of endometriosis should always be given a continuous progestogen with her estrogen replacement to decrease the risk of recurrence.

2. **A history of adenomyosis automatically excludes you from MHT.** FALSE. MHT could cause bleeding and pain with a history of adenomyosis when the uterus is intact. It is not contraindicated, but the doctor should proceed with caution and always give a progestogen. After hysterectomy, there is no documented issue.

3. **A family history of heart disease, liver disease, or breast cancer** *automatically* **excludes you from MHT.** FALSE. The latest research and expert consensus challenge the notion that family history alone should disqualify a woman from MHT candidacy.

4. **Concerns over an increased risk of clotting should automatically exclude you from using MHT.** FALSE. There is nuance here between venous blood clots (like those found in deep venous thrombosis or pulmonary embolism) and arteriolar clotting (like those found in certain strokes). For venous clotting, the use of oral estrogen is well established to increase the risk in DVT in high-dose ORAL formulations containing estrogen. However, nonoral formulations like transdermal or transmucosal formulations do not increase the risk of clotting due to these formulations avoiding the first-pass effect of the liver. Arteriolar clotting is usually due to "sticky platelets" and is slightly increased in any systemic form of estrogen. It is important to note here that in the WHI, no increase in risk in arteriolar clotting was seen among women who started HRT within the 10-year window of the last menstrual period.

5. **A history of migraine headaches automatically excludes you from using MHT.** FALSE. There is no increased risk of stroke with the use of MHT in any form in a patient with a history of migraine without aura. If a patient has a history of migraine with aura—the conversation is more nuanced. The Centers for Disease Control and Prevention (CDC) and World Health Organization (WHO) guidelines recommend that women with migraine with aura not use combined hormone contraception and advise caution when prescribing combined hormone contraception to women with migraine without aura due to the very slight but present increased risk of ischemic stroke, especially in women who smoke. A similar contraindication has not been identified for those with migraine who need HT doses for treatment of symptoms of menopause and/or their headaches, as the doses are much lower for MHT than for contraception.

The decision to embark on MHT should always be based on your unique medical history, risk factors, and symptoms. And your healthcare provider should be consulting current research and clinical guidelines to help ensure you're getting the most up-to-date recommendations. For far too long, women have been denied access to the most effective treatment for menopausal symptoms on the basis of misconceptions and misinformation. We deserve and can demand better!

Hormone Therapy Use After Cancer Treatment— or If You Are a BRCA Carrier

If you are a cancer survivor or a known carrier of the BRCA mutations, I know the consideration of hormone therapy can come with a lot of questions and fears around the presence or resurgence of cancer risk. I also know it can be challenging to get a physician to even have a conversation with you about MHT; the discussion often gets shut down immediately because many healthcare providers don't have the proper knowledge or training on the topic.

Here's what a menopausal woman who's recovered from cancer should be told about MHT: "Having had cancer is a special circumstance, but it's not a universal or automatic contraindication for hormone therapy." And then, the guidance should come from the most up-to-date science available related to your specific type and stage of cancer and your current medication use.

In recent years, the research around the safety of MHT after cancer has been promising. In 2020, the British Menopause Society released findings based on an evaluation of updated science on hormone therapy use after certain types of cancer. The evidence reviewed suggested no increase in risk of recurrence with MHT in women with early-stage endometrial cancer; squamous cell carcinoma of the cervix or adenocarcinoma of the cervix (cervical cancer); or vaginal or vulval cancer. Evidence also showed no adverse effect on survival rates with hormone therapy in women with epithelial ovarian cancer. On women with a history of breast cancer, their conclusion was that it should be a contraindication to the use of systemic MHT.

Considering that breast cancer is one of the most common cancers among women, I know there may be a lot of you who read that last sentence and sighed, screamed, or sobbed; it can feel doubly insulting to be denied an opportunity to relieve symptoms of menopause after enduring cancer treatments. And this is why I want to point out a later analysis published in 2022, which was based on an evaluation of over eight thousand Danish postmenopausal breast cancer survivors who used various types of hormone therapy. For this study, researchers looked at women who had been treated specifically for early-stage estrogen receptor–positive breast cancer. They concluded that neither vaginal estrogen nor MHT was associated with increased risk of recurrence or mortality. They did, however, find an increased risk of recurrence, but not mortality, in those who used vaginal estrogen while taking aromatase inhibitors (sometimes used in the treatment of hormone-receptive breast cancer).

I share these conflicting outcomes not to confuse you but to emphasize the extreme importance of getting access to a menopausal specialist who is following and practicing medicine based on the evolving science on hormone therapy use after breast cancer recovery. Again, the decision of whether to use hormone therapy will require careful consideration of the type and stage of cancer treated and current medication use.

If you are a carrier of the BRCA1 and BRCA2 mutations, you have likely also received either a hard no or conflicting information on the topic of your potential use of MHT. If you're not familiar with BRCA1 and BRCA2, these are genetic mutations that increase the risk of developing breast and ovarian cancer. The data in this area looks at BRCA carriers in two groups: (1) those who have had a prophylactic removal of both ovaries, referred to as a risk-reducing bilateral salpingo-oophorectomy (RRBSO), and (2) those who have not had an RRBSO.

In individuals who've had an RRBSO, research has shown *no increased risk* of breast cancer with MHT use. Since RRBSOs may be recommended to women at a young age—between thirty-five and forty years in BRCA1 and forty to forty-five years in BRCA2—hormone therapy can be especially important to help reduce risk of chronic diseases, such as osteoporosis and heart disease, that can develop as a result of low estrogen. If you have not had an RRBSO, you should discuss your options with your doctor.

The Possible Side Effects of MHT
(and Some Strategies That May Help)

Let's say after a discussion with your healthcare provider and careful consideration of your unique health history, the choice is made—you are ready to start hormone therapy. What's next? First off, I'm sorry to say that you won't experience instant relief of your symptoms. That will come in time, usually after about four weeks, but each individual's response may be different. And remember that you may need to adjust dosage, delivery system, or timing before you find the most effective protocol for you.

One thing you may notice more immediately is certain side effects. I counsel my patients thoroughly on this possibility, but many are still surprised or concerned when side effects arise. Let's look at some of the potential side effects and strategies for managing them.

Potential Side Effects of Estrogen Therapy or Estrogen-Progestogen Therapy

What follows is a selective list. You will find comprehensive lists of side effects in the literature that comes with each prescribed medication. For compounded medication, you will need to ask the pharmacist.

More common side effects are:

- unscheduled uterine bleeding (starting or returning)

- breast tenderness (sometimes enlargement)

Less common side effects are:

- nausea

- abdominal bloating

- fluid retention in extremities

- changes in the shape of the cornea (sometimes leading to contact lens intolerance)

- headache (sometimes migraine)

- dizziness

- mood changes with estrogen-progestogen therapy, particularly with a progestin (synthetic)

- angioedema (swelling, most common in the eyes, lips, and labia)

- gallstones, pancreatitis

Unscheduled bleeding isn't something anyone knowingly wants to sign up for, but it is common—40 percent of patients have unscheduled bleeding after beginning MHT, and it is the number one reason I get calls from my own patients. I reassure them that it is to be expected and quite normal; we are simply "waking up" tissue that has been sleeping for a while. The good news about this common side effect is that it usually resolves on its own, although in some cases strategies to manage it may be helpful (see below). If persistent unscheduled bleeding goes beyond four to six months from the start of hormone therapy, this warrants a pelvic ultrasound to assess the endometrial cavity and, when appropriate, an endometrial biopsy and/or hysteroscopy.

Management of Side Effects

If you experience side effects, some strategies may help. Obviously, changes in medication and/or dosage will require consulting with your doctor or prescribing provider.

For fluid retention, try: restricting salt; ensuring adequate water intake; exercising; taking a mild prescription diuretic.

For bloating, try: switching to low-dose *nonoral* continuous estrogen; lowering the progestogen dose to a level that still protects the uterus; switching to another progestin or to micronized progesterone.

For breast tenderness, try: lowering the estrogen dose; switching to another estrogen; restricting salt; switching to another progestin; cutting down on caffeine and chocolate.

For headache, try: switching to nonoral continuous estrogen; lowering the dose of estrogen or progestogen or both; switching to a continuous-combined regimen; switching to progesterone or a 19-norpregnane derivative; ensuring adequate water intake; restricting salt, caffeine, and alcohol.

For mood changes, try: investigating preexisting depression or anxiety with your clinician or therapist; lowering the progestogen dose; switching to another progestogen or to micronized progesterone; switching from systemic progestin to the progestin intrauterine system; changing to a continuous-combined estrogen-progestogen regimen; ensuring adequate water intake; restricting salt, caffeine, and alcohol.

For nausea, try: in oral estrogen use, taking tablets with meals or before bed; switching to another oral estrogen; switching to nonoral estrogen; lowering estrogen or progestogen dose.

For bleeding, try: lowering the dose of estrogen or increasing progestogen, or switching to a nonprogestogen combined formulation. Note: Currently the only combined formulation available is Duavee, which is a SERM and can be expensive because there's no generic version available.

Choose Your Own Adventure, the Menopause Edition

Congratulations–you have reached the end of the chapter on hormone therapy! *Phew.* I know it was a lot, and I truly hope it was loaded with information you can use to better navigate your own personal journey into menopause and beyond.

I suspect at the end of this chapter you may be in one of two groups, and I suggest moving forward in the book depending on which group you're in:

GROUP 1: You're ready to consult your healthcare provider on how to get started with MHT. If you are in this group, I recommend reading the next chapter as it will help you get what you need from your doctor to get started with MHT. Then be sure to look at the Tool Kit for additional strategies that will support you.

GROUP 2: You have realized hormone therapy is not for you, either because you have a contraindication or because you simply don't want to use it. If you are in this group, you can skim over the MHT-specific questions and resources for your doctor mentioned in the next chapter, but the majority of the chapter will still be relevant for you—especially the section starting on page 129 called How to Make the Most of Your Annual Exam as Your Hormones Change—don't skip this! In the Tool Kit, you will also find dozens of nonhormonal interventions that can help you alleviate symptoms and reduce health risks that come with the diminished hormone levels that are the hallmark of the menopausal transition.

In either case, you have options for action. The sooner you implement hormonal and/or nonhormonal strategies, the sooner you will be able to experience relief from symptoms, and the better your body and mind will be at adapting to the changes that come with menopause.

CHAPTER 8

Preparing for Your Appointment

I prepared for menopause. I really did. But apparently it was never going to matter. No matter how much inner work, organic food, activity, or reduction of stress, perimenopause was going to take me down. I know people who all but breezed through it. I am not one of those people. I'm fifty-one and still having periods. Over the last five years, I have become a shell of who I once was. I've gained forty-five pounds and I cannot lose it no matter what I do. I've taken a variety of natural supplements to help the ever-increasing and worsening symptoms such as fatigue (not even the right word for how exhausted I am), lack of desire for anything, low mood and mood changes, inability to concentrate and brain fog, joint and body pain, hot flashes and night sweats, intermittent insomnia, and let's not forget the identity crisis. After devoting my life to my children and helping others, this is my reward?

—Jody P.

I wrote *The New Menopause* in the hope that it would become an invaluable resource for all things having to do with menopause. But I have to admit that the book does have its limitations—namely that it can't be a replacement for the doctor or healthcare provider who will ultimately (and hopefully) provide the clinical support you need during perimenopause and menopause. Having a healthcare provider who listens to you and stays with you through the menopausal transition is critical!

Unfortunately, I know how difficult it can be to find the medical support that's needed at this stage of life because so many of you have told me so. You've been dismissed and denied a discussion on and access to effective treatments for symptoms. I also know that this experience may have left you feeling defeated, but what if I told you that starting right now, you can begin to envision a different outcome? You can see yourself entering an appointment equipped with the powerful information you'll find in this chapter and exiting with a plan for achieving symptom improvement. Can you see it? It's possible! I'll make sure you have everything you need to help make this vision a reality.

First Things First: Finding the Best Menopause Care Provider

If you already have a relationship with a provider you trust, you may not need the information in this section and you can jump to "How to Prepare for Your Appointment" on page 120, where I address how to talk to your doctor about your therapeutic options, including MHT.

Before you rush off, though, I do want to point out that even if you have trust in and comfort with a doctor, they might not be best equipped to give you the care you need now. Your dependable GP who is your go-to for a bad sore throat or stomach bug? They might not be well read on your changing needs. And the amazing ob-gyn who delivered your baby and performed surgeries and served you very well for twenty years may have received little to no training in menopause care, and may have had no time to become an expert in the area. I know this is true because I *was* that ob-gyn, and I fully admit that for years I was not an informed menopause provider. I relied on my education and training in medical school and residency, and that was just not enough. All this is to say that it's okay to part ways with your doctor and seek out someone who can better support your current healthcare needs at this time in your life.

PLEASE SHARE!

If you have a confirmed and awesome provider of quality menopausal care, I hope you will consider visiting thepauselife.com and our recommended physician database, where you can recommend your doctor's practice to our unbiased referral program. This way, others in your area who may be looking for a provider will discover the recommendation.

If you don't have a healthcare provider currently, I have some suggestions on how you can find a practitioner of menopause care who might be a good fit. If possible, it's best to begin this search with the goal of finding a doctor whom you can see in person. In-person visits allow providers to physically assess your overall health, and the appointments can be much more efficient since the doctor can provide specialized treatment or screenings on demand. Plus, in-person care can make it easier to communicate your questions and concerns, get immediate feedback, and help you establish a good doctor-patient relationship. However, even as I stress this importance, I know the reality is that in some regions specialized care is limited and you may need to connect virtually to a provider. And the truth is, if you find a virtual doctor who listens to you and respects you as a patient, that's far better than a doctor who dismisses you in person!

Here are the steps to take to find a provider:

1. Consider insurance coverage. If you have health insurance and you plan or hope to use your insurance coverage, you will want to see what "in-network" providers are available to you. Most insurance companies offer a search feature that will allow you to input your region and the specialty you are seeking. Unfortunately, menopause care is not a commonly listed category, so you'll be best served by searching for an ob-gyn and, if you identify one who may work, calling to see if they have any experience treating menopausal women. If you can't find an in-network provider, check with your insurance company to determine your out-of-network benefits.

2. Consult my Recommended Physicians list. The list of recommended physicians that I keep on my website has been built by submissions and testimonials from people worldwide who have had an exceptional experience that they want to share. I do not personally know the doctors on the list, but my team does their due diligence in verifying each referral listed (we confirm that they are in practice and confirm contact information). If you don't find any providers listed in your area, you can also visit the Menopause Society website menopause.org, and their "Find a Menopause Practitioner" database to find a local provider. However you identify a potential candidate, it's still a good idea to call and make sure that they are willing to discuss menopause and all of your therapeutic options.

3. **Ask your doctor for a referral.** If you came to your general practitioner or gynecologist with severe back pain or terrible headaches, they would likely refer you to a specialist—an orthopedist or a neurologist respectively. It should be no different with symptoms of menopause! Ideally, your present healthcare provider will recognize the gap in their knowledge and will be willing to help you find someone who specializes in what you need.

4. **Ask people you know for a referral.** Many people feel most comfortable visiting a physician who is recommended by someone they know. Ask your friends, family members, neighbors, or coworkers if they (or anyone they know) can recommend a provider for menopausal care. You can also check local Facebook groups for suggestions.

5. **Consider virtual menopause care.** If you can't find a local-ish practitioner, you may be able to find someone you can work with via telemedicine. Thankfully, an increasing number of healthcare providers are offering this option, which allows increased access to quality care. You can also check Evernow and Alloy Health for options. See the resources section on page 257 for contact information.

How to Prepare for Your Appointment

When researchers from Yale University looked at over five hundred thousand insurance claims from women in various stages of menopause, they found that three hundred thousand of the claims were related to patients seeking medical assistance for significant menopausal symptoms—and that 75 percent of the patients left without treatment. I share this insight for a couple reasons—first, because it makes me want to scream profanities and shout, "*Why?*" (and then have my husband peek his head in and say, "What now?"); second, because it's evidence that if you're feeling frustrated trying to find relief from your menopausal symptoms, you're certainly not alone; and third, because it demonstrates how you should approach your appointment—you need more than just questions and details of your struggles; you need to be prepared with a strategy.

The best strategy for success with your doctor's appointment involves having a plan in the areas of timing and information.

Timing

- CONSIDER GETTING AHEAD OF MENOPAUSAL SYMPTOMS. In pregnancy, there's a specific medical appointment referred to as a "prepregnancy" visit. The purpose of this visit is to help establish care, review what the options are, and get educated about what to expect. There's no equivalent "premenopause" visit—but can you imagine how life-changing it could be if there was one as a standard part of women's healthcare? I have noticed a trend in my patients who have decided not to wait for this to become standard and are coming in to get a plan in place. They want to "get ahead of things" before the onset of symptoms and take any preventative measures possible. It's a radical idea that I am 100 percent on board with.

- GET AN EARLY APPOINTMENT. I recommend trying to schedule the first appointment of the morning to ensure a fresh physician. I know this may sound like a small thing, but doctors are humans too, and their energy and attention can drag as the day goes. You may get the best version of your doctor if you see them in the morning.

- ACKNOWLEDGE THE NATURE OF YOUR APPOINTMENT. When you call to make your appointment, tell the staff you have issues you would like to discuss, so the scheduler knows to block off additional time if time is available. Don't expect a menopause visit to be covered in a "Well Woman Exam"—that is a screening exam for things like breast and cervical cancer and common chronic illnesses, *not* for menopause. Make it clear that you need a "problem visit" to ensure that you get the most amount of time allotted for this discussion.

- SHOW UP IN A FASTED STATE. Depending on the time of your appointment (hopefully early), consider showing up in a fasted state (no food/drink other than water after midnight). This way if your doctor wants to run tests that require you to have fasted, you can get them run right then and there rather than having to come back another time.

Information

FAMILY HISTORY

Write down your family history of diseases and illnesses, which relative had them, and at what age. This is information that your provider will ask for, and having it written out in advance will save time and give them the notes they need for their files. And, importantly, this information could qualify you for certain medical tests you may not otherwise be qualified for. For example, if you have fatigue *and* a family history of hypothyroidism, your physician can utilize that diagnostic code and increase your chances of insurance covering the test. Your family history can also determine if you are a candidate for certain hormone therapies.

SYMPTOM JOURNAL

If you haven't already, start keeping a symptom journal of any noticeable changes to your health. Make note of any new aches and pains, increases in fatigue, gastrointestinal issues, differences in hair or skin, weight gain or loss, mental health or memory challenges, and so on. Be as detailed as you can—your doctor will want to know how long you've been experiencing the symptoms and if they've become more or less severe. See Appendix C, page 264, for a sample of this kind of journal—and use this allotted space as a start to your own recordkeeping.

A SENSE OF YOUR PERSONAL PREFERENCES

Think about your preferences for managing your symptoms and long-term health. Do you want to consider hormone therapy or would you prefer a nonhormonal approach? Do you want recommended lifestyle modifications? Consider your goals and how you'd like to get there, and be ready to share the specifics with your healthcare provider. You want to be prepared to advocate for yourself while at the same time making it clear that you are asking your provider for their professional medical opinion based on your medical history. How your doctor responds to this invitation for a collaborative practitioner-patient relationship should tell you a lot about your chances for getting the care you want from them.

Here are some questions to ask that may help you get aligned with the right practitioner (the answers provided may also help you further refine your personal menopausal care preferences).

Can you share your experience and training prescribing MHT? How familiar are you with the latest research and guidelines?

Have you successfully treated patients with symptoms similar to mine using MHT? Can you provide specific examples?

How do you stay updated on advancements and new studies in the field of menopause and hormone therapy?

Are you open to discussing and considering alternative or complementary therapies alongside MHT to optimize my treatment plan?

How do you approach managing potential side effects of MHT and what steps do you take to minimize associated risks?

Are you open to exploring different forms of MHT based on patient preferences, and how do you tailor treatment plans to individual lifestyles?

How do you support patients who may be interested in transitioning from other healthcare providers for their MHT needs?

If, by shared decision making, we decide that I am not a candidate for MHT, how will you manage my menopause?

UPDATED SCIENTIFIC INSIGHT ON THE USE OF MENOPAUSAL HORMONE THERAPY

I don't mean to put the responsibility of providing scientific evidence on you, the patient, but it's in your own best interest to be prepared with some key bits of information. Here's why: Few doctors have received formal training in menopause medicine, and it's likely in most cases that the yearly requirements for recertification established by the medical society board (for example, the American Board of Obstetrics and Gynecology) have not included updated science on menopause as part of your physician's annual education requirement. This is especially true when it comes to the latest information on menopausal hormone therapy. In other words, you may need to help your healthcare provider so that they can help you.

Most healthcare practitioners today are exhausted and overworked, and they're also under intense pressure to keep appointments to fifteen minutes or less. You'll want to keep this in mind when you go in for your appointment. Maybe you will have underlined or highlighted some of the information in this book and can present it to your new doctor. Or see below for updated statements and statistics on the use of menopausal hormone therapy, as well as a very helpful menopause questionnaire. I have reiterated these key, helpful pieces of information in Appendix A (statements and stats) and B (questionnaire) so you can cut them out of the book if you don't want to bring the whole book to your appointment. Either way, be ready to say: "Here's some info from credible sources on the use of hormone therapy in menopausal women. I hope we can work together to determine the most appropriate course of treatment for my symptoms."

Updated Statements and Stats on the Use of Menopausal Hormone Therapy

In 2022, **the North American Menopause Society (NAMS)**, now the Menopause Society, issued an updated position on hormone therapy, "The 2022 Hormone Therapy Position Statement of the North American Menopause Society" (*Menopause.* 2022;29[7]:767-794. doi: 10.1097/GME .0000000000002028), with the consensus being that for healthy people born female younger than sixty, and within ten years of menopause onset, the benefits of hormone therapy outweigh the risks. This update was a significant rewrite of their prior recommendation, which said that MHT was recommended only for severe symptoms and at the lowest dose for the shortest time.

In 2020, **the American Heart Association** published "Menopause Transition and Cardiovascular Disease Risk: Implications for Timing of Early Prevention: A Scientific Statement from the American Heart Association" (*Circulation.* 2020;142[25]:e506-e532. doi:10.1161/CIR.0000000000000912). This statement acknowledged the accelerated increase in cardiovascular risk brought about by the menopausal transition and emphasized the importance of early intervention strategies to help reduce this risk. The findings noted that those who are treated with hormone therapy along with a comprehensive nutrition and lifestyle approach have lower cardiovascular risks and lesser likelihood of negative disease outcomes.

The US Food and Drug Administration has approved MHT to treat four conditions associated with menopause:

1. **Vasomotor symptoms:** includes hot flashes, night sweats, heart palpitations, and sleep disturbances

2. **Bone loss:** includes weakening bones and osteoporosis

3. **Premature hypoestrogenism (estrogen deficiency):** as a result of menopause or premature menopause resulting from surgery such as oophorectomy (with or without hysterectomy), or radiation or chemotherapy

4. **Genitourinary symptoms:** includes frequent urination, burning with urination, recurrent urinary tract infections, vaginal dryness, pain with intercourse

Additionally, research (see chapter 8 references for study citations) has shown that hormone therapy can help improve and relieve symptoms related to the following conditions:

- SARCOPENIA (DECREASED MUSCLE MASS): Hormone therapy can counteract sarcopenia related to aging, a decrease in estrogen production, and the transition to menopause.

- COGNITION: When initiated immediately after hysterectomy with bilateral oophorectomy, estrogen therapy may provide some cognitive benefit.

- SKIN AND HAIR CONDITIONS: These include thinning hair and skin, increased bruising, and loss of skin elasticity.

- JOINT PAIN: Women participating in several studies have reported less joint pain or stiffness with hormone therapy compared with placebo.

- DIABETES: While not FDA approved for treatment of type 2 diabetes, MHT in otherwise healthy women with preexisting type 2 diabetes may improve glycemic control when used to manage menopause symptoms.

- DEPRESSION: While not FDA approved for the treatment of depression, estrogen-based therapies may complement clinical response to antidepressants in midlife and older women when prescribed to treat menopausal symptoms.

The Greene Scale: Another Way to Help Your Doctor Help You

Along with the updated MHT info above, you can also complete the Greene Scale questionnaire in advance of an appointment with a menopausal healthcare provider. This symptom checker was first created in 1976 but has been updated since, and it is still widely used as a tool for helping identify treatment needs during the menopausal transition.

On the Menopause Symptom Scoring Sheet below, score each symptom 1 for mild, 2 for moderate, 3 for severe, and 0 if you do not have that particular symptom.

SYMPTOM	SCORE
Hot Flashes	_____
Lightheaded Feelings	_____
Headaches	_____
Irritability	_____
Depression	_____
Unloved Feelings	_____
Anxiety	_____
Mood Changes	_____
Sleeplessness	_____
Unusual Tiredness	_____
Backache	_____
Joint Pain	_____
Muscle Pain	_____
New Facial Hair	_____
Dry Skin	_____
Crawling Feelings Under the Skin	_____
Less Sexual Feelings	_____
Dry Vagina	_____
Uncomfortable Intercourse	_____
Urinary Frequency	_____
TOTAL	_____

Adapted from Greene JG. Constructing a standard climacteric standard. Maturitas 1998;29:25-31.

A score of 15 or over usually indicates that estrogen deficiency is likely contributing to your symptoms, and in my practice this means we begin the discussion of therapy immediately. Scores of 20–50 are common in symptomatic women, and with adequate treatment tailored to you, your score should reduce to 10 or under in three to six months.

Red Flags That Suggest Your Search for the Right Provider Might Not Be Over

I wish I could say that once you've done the work to find a healthcare provider and you've prepared for your appointment, everything else is just going to go perfectly, but I can't promise you this. The reality is that the outcome of your appointment is unpredictable. I hope for your sake it goes well, but there are a few things that I would consider signs of it *not* having gone well. If you hear any of the following, I would consider continuing your search for the right provider:

- "SORRY, IT'S JUST THE TIME OF YOUR LIFE." Yes, menopause is a natural stage, but that does not mean you have to endure the symptoms of it without help. Other similarly unacceptable phrases might be "It's just your new normal" and "You're going to have to deal with it." Move on.

- "I DON'T PRESCRIBE MHT." It's also unacceptable for your healthcare provider to tell you that they don't prescribe hormone therapy. Ultimately, the choice is up to you, and at the very least you deserve a discussion about whether the benefits outweigh the risks for you and your personal medical history. It should always be a nuanced conversation; it should never be a flat-out "No." If they continue to refuse, remember to check out our Recommended Physicians database (https://thepauselife.com/pages/recommended-physicians) to find a new provider, or you can reference the Menopause Society Certified Practitioners database (https://portal.menopause.org/NAMS /NAMS/Directory/Menopause-Practitioner.aspx) to find a provider in your area.

- "I'LL ONLY PRESCRIBE HORMONE THERAPY FOR A SPECIFIC TIME FRAME."
  Do not allow your provider to impose unnecessary time restrictions:
  for example, only prescribing it once or for a year or two. It's
  responsible medicine to insist on monitoring adverse side effects of a
  prescribed medication, but the conversation on the duration of MHT
  use should be an ongoing one. If your symptoms persist, you'll still
  need help to manage them.

How to Make the Most of Your Annual Exam as Your Hormones Change

I hope you are getting your annual physical. These yearly checkups are
intended to screen you for a set list of common diseases and conditions,
and they are important. You can get an annual exam from your general
practitioner or ask your menopause provider if it makes sense to have
them perform this yearly screening. In either case, you make the most of
the appointment by understanding a little about the purpose of the standard blood tests that are run, and by considering some add-on tests that
are important to check in menopause.

Standard Blood Tests (and Add-Ons to Ask For)

A note on potential costs and insurance coverage: A screening visit and
the blood tests that go along with it are almost always covered by insurance, but it's really hard to predict what add-ons may be covered. Some
companies won't pay for anything that's outside of what they've prenego-
tiated as part of the screening exam, but others will be more liberal. For
this reason, you may want to request some of the add-on lab work during
your problem visit that's specific to menopausal symptoms—insurance
companies are more likely to cover labs related to specific symptoms and
history—rather than during your annual exam. (I wish I could offer more
universal guidance in this area, but insurance is so wildly variable these
days.)

COMPLETE BLOOD COUNT (CBC), COMPREHENSIVE METABOLIC
PANEL (CMP), AND LIPID PANEL

These three tests are standard screening tests that do not require symptoms for insurance to cover them during an annual exam.

A *complete blood count (CBC)* test is one that measures and counts all your blood cells, including red blood cells, white blood cells, platelets, hemoglobin, and hematocrit. The results of this test can be used to diagnose underlying infections, which can cause a high or low white blood cell count; leukemia or lymphoma; anemia; or certain vitamin deficiencies.

A *comprehensive metabolic panel (CMP)* reveals details about your metabolic, liver, and kidney function. The CMP test checks electrolytes, such as sodium, calcium, and potassium; albumin; blood urea nitrogen; carbon dioxide; chloride; creatinine; glucose; total bilirubin and protein; and liver enzymes.

A *lipid panel* (drawn while fasting) will measure your HDL ("good") cholesterol, LDL ("bad") cholesterol, and triglycerides. These are cholesterol levels that will provide a picture of your overall heart health, and your doctor will review and discuss the specifics of your test results with you. If you want to go a little further, you can use the results from your lab work to calculate your HDL-to-triglycerides ratio. According to a study published in the *Journal of the American Heart Association,* this ratio may be a good predictor of major adverse cardiovascular events in women, and especially in postmenopausal women. To calculate your HDL-to-triglycerides ratio, simply divide your triglyceride level by your HDL level in mg/dL (or mmol/L), then compare your answer to the scale below:

IDEAL: 2.0 or less
GOOD: 4.0 to 6.0
BAD: over 6.0 or above

If your ratio is ranked ideal or good, keep checking your ratio each time you get your cholesterol levels run. If it's bad, be sure to discuss it with your doctor as soon as possible. You can also start applying the nutritional changes and other strategies listed in the Tool Kit entry "High Cholesterol/ High Triglycerides" (see page 197).

Ask for These Add-Ons: Lipoprotein (a) and Apolipoprotein B, aka Lp(a) and ApoB.

ApoB and Lp(a) are two important markers that healthcare professionals check to assess your risk of heart disease, and they are especially important if your HDL-to-triglycerides ratio is in the "bad" score range.

Let me explain in simple terms why it's important to have these checked.

ApoB is a protein found in your blood that is responsible for carrying cholesterol to various parts of your body, including your arteries. High levels of ApoB are associated with an increased risk of atherosclerosis, a condition where fatty deposits build up in your arteries, potentially leading to heart disease and stroke. By checking your ApoB levels, your doctor can get a *more accurate measure* of the harmful cholesterol in your blood than just measuring LDL cholesterol alone. This can help in assessing your risk of heart disease more accurately.

Lp(a) is a type of cholesterol particle in your blood, and high levels of Lp(a) are associated with an increased risk of heart disease, especially when it comes to coronary artery disease. Elevated Lp(a) levels can contribute to the formation of plaques in your arteries, which can lead to heart attacks and other cardiovascular problems. Checking your Lp(a) levels can help identify your genetic predisposition to heart disease.

Having your ApoB and Lp(a) levels checked is important because these provide a more comprehensive assessment of your cardiovascular risk beyond traditional cholesterol tests. Knowing your levels can help your doctor better tailor your treatment plan or lifestyle changes to reduce your risk of heart disease. It's essential to discuss the results with your healthcare provider to understand your individual risk and develop a plan to maintain or improve your heart health.

HEMOGLOBIN A1C (HBA1C)

The HbA1c test measures your average blood sugar over the last two–three months. The higher your HbA1C, the greater your risk for developing type 2 diabetes. A high HbA1C marker may also increase your risk of Alzheimer's disease and cancer.

Ask for This Add-On: If you have a family history of obesity, acanthosis nigricans, or other known risk factors for insulin resistance, you may want to consider asking for the homeostatic model assessment for insulin resistance (HOMA-IR) to be run. HOMA-IR allows a practitioner to assess how responsive you are to insulin by dividing fasting by fasting glucose.

THYROID PANEL

Your annual physical blood work will typically check your thyroid-stimulating hormone or TSH, an important marker of thyroid function. In some cases, however, TSH alone won't allow for an underlying thyroid condition to be identified.

Ask for This Add-On: Ask for a comprehensive thyroid panel that includes TSH and free T4, free T3, reverse T3, and two types of thyroid antibody levels called anti-TPO and anti-thyroglobulin. I definitely recommend you ask for these specific factors to be measured if you are experiencing symptoms such as chronic fatigue, cold intolerance, hair loss, forgetfulness, constipation, unexplained weight gain or loss, or general feelings of depression. Thyroid disorders tend to go undiagnosed for far too long, so be sure to have this comprehensive panel done next time you are at the doctor.

VITAMIN D

Forty-two percent of patients on average have low vitamin D, and this number gets worse with age and menopause. This deficiency can be due to where you live (i.e., limited sun exposure); darker skin, which limits absorption; a genetic issue; an absorption issue; or kidney disease. Low D levels can make you more susceptible to developing osteoporosis, and healthy levels of this crucial nutrient may support immune and heart health.

Ask for These Add-Ons: Zinc and magnesium. Zinc is used by your body in cell production and immune functions. When you're zinc deficient, your body can't produce healthy new cells. This deficiency leads to symptoms such as unexplained weight loss, wounds that won't heal, lack of alertness, and decreased sense of smell and taste.

You'll also want to have your magnesium level checked, as deficiency is linked to poor sleep, nerve problems, mood disorders, fatigue, muscle cramping, headaches, and brittle hair and nails. It is also important for heart health, for blood pressure, and to keep your thyroid in balance.

Nonstandard Blood Tests

The following are not routinely done in all patients as a screening test, but I think they are important and relevant to check in menopause, and any doctor can request them with the check of a couple of boxes on lab requesting paperwork (but again, coverage by insurance may be another issue, and proper documentation is key). I recommend these tests to all my patients at my menopause clinic.

ANEMIA PANEL (IRON, FERRITIN, FOLATE, AND VITAMIN B12)

While the CBC panel will check for anemia, I recommend this more comprehensive panel for women in the menopausal transition. Anemia in menopause is a major cause of chronic fatigue, and chronic fatigue affects over 70 percent of postmenopausal women, so this is important to investigate for all of my patients. Low vitamin B12 is common among vegetarians and vegans but can also exist among omnivores due to nutrient malabsorption issues caused by antibiotic overuse or celiac or Crohn's disease. Low iron can present as anemia or even hypothyroidism. Even if you're not anemic (which can be tested for with a CBC), you can still be iron deficient—which is why testing for iron and ferritin separately is important.

CHRONIC INFLAMMATION TESTING: HIGH-SENSITIVITY C-REACTIVE PROTEIN (HsCRP) AND ERYTHROCYTE SEDIMENTATION RATE

When estrogen levels begin to decline during perimenopause, we start to lose out on its anti-inflammatory effect and the result can often present itself as chronic nonspecific inflammation. You can check and monitor levels of inflammation by testing levels of specific inflammatory markers, such as high-sensitivity c-reactive protein (HsCRP), erythrocyte sedimentation rate, and plasma viscosity. I will suggest that my patients have these markers checked before and about four months after we've implemented any lifestyle modifications. The results allow us to determine how successful any nutrition/diet/supplements/pharmacology interventions were at helping lower these markers.

HsCRP is naturally produced in the liver in response to inflammation. A high level of CRP in your blood can occur due to several inflammatory conditions. The ESR test can also help your doctor identify that inflammation is occurring. Both measures are taken initially to help establish an inflammation baseline, and if a patient needs to implement inflammation-lowering strategies, we can use this baseline to help keep track of improvements. If we are not able to lower these with our interventions, we begin to investigate alternative causes of this elevation.

Remember the Importance of Self-Care

I hope you are able to use the information and tools in this chapter to better advocate for yourself as you seek out quality menopausal healthcare. As you search, I encourage you to also prioritize self-care by focusing on achieving quality sleep, implementing stress-lowering practices, eating an anti-inflammatory diet, and getting regular exercise. While paying attention to these lifestyle strategies isn't guaranteed to reduce all your symptoms, consistency in these areas can produce some relief and will certainly deliver desired health benefits.

Part Three

SYMPTOMS AND SOLUTIONS

CHAPTER 9

The Daily Behaviors That Contribute to Menopause Health

During medical school and throughout my medical career, I was taught that the symptoms likely to be brought on by menopause were hot flashes, night sweats, and genitourinary syndrome. It was also well established that there was an increased risk of osteoporosis. And that was basically it. Talk about a molehill being made out of a mountain—what's clear now, many years later, is that menopause has a potential role in dozens of symptoms and conditions (see page 148).

My generation of medical students and ob-gyn residents received little training in menopause: maybe a one-hour lecture in medical school and another six hours in residency. There were no "menopause clinics," meaning no specialized care training in menopause. And by the end of my residency, we were under the assumption that hormone replacement therapy was dangerous because of the initial findings from the WHI study (see chapter 3 for this discussion).

Every year since my residency, I have completed the continuing medical education required for board certification. Out of the thousands of articles that the American Board of Obstetrics and Gynecology (ABOG) has collected for my review, I can think of only a handful that were specific to menopause. In fact, there is no "menopause" category in our board review sets. Surgery, obstetrics, pediatric gynecology, and ethics all are covered—but there is no specific category for menopause.

To be honest, I now realize that I was a terrible menopause provider for years. I completely relied on what was put forth to me by ABOG, and I thought I was well prepared for taking care of a woman in menopause. While I am incredibly proud of what I did learn in my ob-gyn training, I now know that there were huge gaps in my knowledge concerning the optimal health of the menopausal woman.

My understanding of menopause began to change when three things happened practically all at once: I started going through menopause; my patients started to go through menopause in droves (we were roughly the same age); and I began talking about menopause on social media. I noticed an uptick in seemingly unexplained symptoms and changes to my health. My cholesterol suddenly increased, despite no changes in my diet and exercise. My joint pain became nearly debilitating without injury. And my fatigue was interfering with my life. I noticed that many of my patients were complaining of the same things, and as I began sharing about my symptoms on social media, I started getting thousands of comments saying, "Me too!"

I had no idea that my increasing cholesterol, joint pain, and fatigue could be related to menopause. My followers would also ask if a certain condition could possibly be related to menopausal hormone changes. Things like frozen shoulder, vertigo, TMJ . . . "Could these possibly have anything to do with menopause?" The questions kept coming, and I began to see patterns emerging. In an effort to help and to fulfill my own medical curiosity, I began doing deep dives into the recent scientific literature and finding clear evidence that, yes, in a lot of cases, there was a link. I was shocked. Remember, I had not been taught that menopause was more than the "classic symptoms." I had also been taught that women tend to somaticize, or convert their psychological symptoms into physical ones. Yet there was clear evidence of the links between symptoms and diseases in multiple organ systems. And this was not common knowledge, nor were these facts being disseminated through the usual continuing-education channels for people in my specialty.

Identifying evidence of a link is one thing, but it's another thing altogether to find research that has determined that a specific treatment for a symptom of menopause is effective. For the Menopause Tool Kit (beginning on page 147), I've spent countless hours in the latter area, digging into the science of solutions, or potential ones at least. What I found is that for some symptoms there is clear evidence that specific treatments might be helpful or preventative. For example, migraine headaches and body composition changes have been extensively studied in the context of menopause, so the Tool Kit recommendations are robust. Symptoms such as tinnitus and asthma, on the other hand, have only recently emerged as related to menopause, so the conclusions aren't as concrete. For these, I've consulted specialty websites for aspects of treatment. In many of these areas, we need a lot more research. Thankfully unprecedented interest and attention are now being paid to menopause—and hopefully this will translate to a greater investment in the scientific study of menopause, and in turn an ever-improving ability to treat symptoms that can cause so much suffering.

One point that became clear after reviewing hundreds of studies is that there are universal truths about how we create good health after menopause. The first truth: Good menopausal health is not an accident. And the second: It is never, ever going to be achieved as the result of a single pill or supplement or treatment. It is instead the result of adopting a collection of daily behaviors and habits that many of us may have previously neglected (or that we just "got away with" being inconsistent about in our younger years). These daily behaviors focus on what are the key components of the Menopause Tool Kit: nutrition, exercise, pharmacology, and supplementation. If you can pay attention to these areas of your life and within them create positive, health-enriching patterns, you will go a long way toward improving your quality of life during the menopausal transition and beyond. You will also reduce risk of chronic disease down the road. Let's look a little closer at each of these key components.

Anti-Inflammatory Nutrition

A core foundation of the Menopause Tool Kit is anti-inflammatory nutrition. As estrogen levels decline during the menopausal transition, you lose an incredibly valuable ally in the fight against inflammation. You can compensate somewhat for this loss by being highly strategic about what you eat. Anti-inflammatory nutrition means eating healthy fats, lean meats, and antioxidant-rich fruits and vegetables, and increasing your fiber intake. It also means limiting intake of alcohol, processed meats, and processed foods generally. When you eat this way most of the time, you can reduce many symptoms and side effects of menopause like weight gain, bone loss, and the risk of chronic diseases such as heart disease and type 2 diabetes.

Strength- and Endurance-Building Exercise

Exercise can deliver unparalleled improvements to cardiovascular, metabolic, and mental health, making it essential to taking care of yourself no matter what stage of life you are in. In menopause, decreasing hormone levels lead to both muscle and bone loss, so your focus with exercise is to work strategically to counteract this effect. You must exercise to increase and preserve muscle and strength (not to achieve some idealized version of your "skinny" self). The best exercise for you, then, is resistance training, which should include lifting weights and completing simple functional movements using your own body weight. It's also important to get plenty of aerobic exercise, such as walking, jogging, and/or running to encourage respiratory and cardiovascular endurance as you age.

Cardio + Resistance Training: An Unbeatable Combination

Aerobic training, aka cardio, is exercise that involves continuous, rhythmic movements that elevate heart rate and breathing. There are a lot of potential cardio options, including running, cycling, swimming, dancing, rowing, boxing, and more (this means if you haven't found a cardio exercise you like, consider trying a different type). Aerobic training has been shown to be particularly effective in helping reduce the accumulation of fat, which we are more susceptible to in menopause.

You get an even greater benefit when you do both cardio and resistance training. This combination provides the fat-loss benefits of aerobic training and the muscle-building effects of resistance training, the best for healthy body composition. Lifting weights or performing exercises like push-ups can promote muscle gain, which can help counteract the natural age-related decline in muscle mass and metabolism. For an excellent book on the subject, read *Forever Strong* by Dr. Gabrielle Lyon.

Evidence-Based Pharmacology

Pharmacology refers to treatments that your healthcare provider can prescribe or recommend to reduce symptoms such as hot flashes, night sweats, bone loss, premature estrogen deficiency, and genitourinary issues like vaginal dryness and frequent urination. The primary pharmacological treatment for some, but not all, symptoms of menopause is menopausal hormone therapy. When there is evidence of MHT's effectiveness in reducing or eliminating a symptom, I will make it clear. I will also point out when there simply isn't enough research to recommend it as part of your approach to pursuing relief for a specific symptom. If you are not a candidate for hormone therapy (visit chapter 7 to determine if it may be right for you), there are other medications and supplements available that can be very effective in treating your symptoms. When it comes to pharmacological treatments, it is essential that you meet with your menopause-educated provider to review your symptoms, goals, and family history so that they can help you identify the best and safest methods for you.

Strategic Supplementation

Throughout the Tool Kit, you will find that some of the strategies for your symptoms include the use of certain supplements. Supplements can play a very important role in supporting your health, especially when specific nutrients are lacking or when certain health goals require extra support. And if you have a known clinical deficiency, you will want your healthcare provider to help prescribe proper supplement dosages to help correct this deficiency. However, supplements should never be used as a replacement for a diet rich in fruits, vegetables, lean proteins, whole grains, and healthy fats. This is because there's simply no pill or powder that can replicate the full spectrum of nutrients, fiber, and health benefits that you can get from food.

I do want to point out that taking high doses of supplements will not give you any superpowers against a disease linked to a deficiency. For example, vitamin C deficiency harms the immune system, but taking large doses will not give you more resistance against disease. I know that some alternative practitioners and supplement companies make plenty of claims that megadosing is some kind of miracle cure, but this simply isn't true (although they may be perfectly fine with you buying and taking more supplements than you need).

The Importance of Supplement Safety and Purity

Supplements are wildly popular, and this translates to consumers having a lot of choices, which can in turn lead to confusion about how to pick the best options. As a healthcare provider and a supplier of supplements through my own company, I recommend prioritizing products that are high quality, safe, and pure. Here are some key considerations to ensure the quality, safety, and purity of the supplements you choose:

1. *Third-party testing.* Reputable supplement brands invest in third-party testing. These independent laboratories assess the purity and potency of supplements to ensure they meet label claims.

2. *Transparency.* Trustworthy brands are transparent about their sourcing, manufacturing processes, and quality control measures. You should be able to easily access information about where the ingredients come from, how they are processed, and what steps are taken to prevent contamination.

3. *Avoid proprietary blends.* Some supplements hide behind proprietary blends, which group ingredients together without specifying indi-

vidual dosages. This lack of transparency makes it impossible to know what you're really consuming. Opt for products with clearly listed ingredient amounts.

4. *Check for allergens.* If you have allergies or sensitivities, carefully read labels to ensure that supplements are free from common allergies like gluten, soy, dairy, or nuts.

Before starting any new supplement regimen, consult with a knowledgeable healthcare provider, especially if you have underlying health conditions or are taking medications. Your doctor or other provider can help you determine which supplements are safe and appropriate for your needs. Of course, you want to make sure the healthcare provider with whom you're working is qualified to offer guidance on supplements (or on any other health-related issue, for that matter). You can check qualifications by verifying their credentials and ensuring that they have a background in healthcare or nutrition and adhere to ethical standards.

In addition to the key components of menopausal health you'll find most represented in the Tool Kit, I have found there are a few other areas of life where practicing good habits can produce profound rewards. These practices include efforts aimed at stress reduction, sleep optimization, and community engagement.

Stress Reduction

Not only does chronic stress downgrade quality of life, it can also lead to high levels of glucocorticoids. Glucocorticoids are stress hormones, such as cortisol, that when elevated can cause and exacerbate the metabolic dysfunction brought on by the hormone shifts of menopause. Stress hormones weaken the immune response, promote high cholesterol, and reduce the use of glucose by your muscle tissues, increasing the risk of high blood sugar, insulin resistance, and type 2 diabetes.

Taking steps to reduce stress may help you avoid some of its metabolic disruption. Stress reduction can also boost mental health, improve overall well-being, and lessen some symptoms of menopause. You may already have identified activities that help lower your stress levels, and the key is to be consistent with their practice. Mindfulness, meditation and breathing, journaling, and yoga are techniques that can help reduce acute stress levels over time. Counseling, such as cognitive behavioral therapy (CBT), can also help, as it encourages you to identify and challenge normative beliefs, allowing you to set realistic expectations and adopt more functional thoughts.

Sleep Optimization

Menopause is a notorious sleep disruptor; it can cause night sweats, restlessness, sleep apnea, or other conditions that interfere with you getting restorative sleep. As with chronic stress, a pattern of poor sleep can contribute to high cortisol levels. It can also increase your risk of developing chronic sleep-related conditions such as sleep apnea and insomnia, which are associated with greater risk of depression, hypertension, type 2 diabetes, heart attack, and stroke. Getting quality sleep during the menopausal transition and beyond does not happen by accident. Some of the most effective ways to encourage a good night's sleep include:

- SETTING THE RIGHT TEMPERATURE. Sleep is best when the temperature is between 60 and 67 degrees. If it's not possible to achieve this temperature range, consider adding a standing fan to your room that can encourage good air circulation.

- GETTING REGULAR EXERCISE. Research has shown that incorporating regular exercise into your life can help you fall asleep faster and increase sleep duration and quality. The timing of exercise may matter—for some people, working out closer to bedtime can make it harder to fall asleep. Pay attention to your own body's response to physical activity as it relates to rest and make adjustments as needed.

- FOCUSING ON SLEEP HYGIENE. This is critical in menopause. You can set yourself up for a good night's sleep by avoiding napping after 3:00 P.M., creating relaxing bedtime rituals, and sticking to a sleep schedule. You'll also get better-quality rest if you avoid heavy meals too close to bedtime and minimize exposure to light, especially the kind that's emitted by our LED TVs and smartphone screens. A good rule of thumb is to keep electronics out of your bedroom.

Community Engagement

Going through menopause can be a very lonely experience, even if you are fortunate enough to have a group of close female friends who are of a similar age. This is because the exact age when perimenopause starts and severity of symptoms can vary a great deal, and your friends might not "get it" until they too are there. Fortunately, social media and other online communities are full of people who do get it, and they are helping each other feel less alone in their journey through menopause and less confused by the seemingly strange symptoms that arise. I offer free access to our 'Pause Life Community, and there are so many other great online spaces out there, including Hey Perry, Stripes, The Swell, and PeloPause. Connecting with others who understand what you're going through and who are willing to have open and honest conversations can provide invaluable validation, information, strategies, friendship, and more.

Menopausal Best Practices

The following pointers constitute a general "starter tool kit" that applies to every woman going through menopause:

NUTRITION

- Consider intermittent fasting for the anti-inflammatory benefits (see more on page 164)

- Utilization of a nutrition tracking mechanism: my favorite is Cronometer*

- Adequate protein intake: at least 1.3–1.6 grams of protein per kilogram of ideal body weight per day

- Less than 25 grams of added sugars per day

- More than 25 grams of fiber per day

MOVEMENT

- Stretching every day

- Balance training every day

- Resistance training: focusing on progressively increasing load three days/week (a push day, a pull day, and a leg day)

- Cardiovascular training (see sidebar page 139)

PHARMACOLOGY

- Consider MHT if for you the benefits outweigh the risks

- Other pharmacology as indicated

SUPPLEMENTATION (IF NOT ABLE TO GET FROM FOOD)

- Fiber intake to surpass 25 grams total per day

- Omega-3 fatty acids, 2 g/day

- Vitamin D, 4,000 IU/day with vitamin K

- Creatine, 5 g/day

---

* Full disclosure: I am an affiliate of Cronometer, and my students who enroll in my online program for the Galveston Diet upgrade to the paid version, but Cronometer also offers a free version.

- Specific collagen peptides with Fortibone for bone strength and Verisol for skin collagen
- Optional: turmeric, berberine, vitamin E based on risk factors/disease

STRESS REDUCTION

- *Sunshine:* Viewing sunlight increases your brain's production of serotonin, the neurotransmitter that's linked to mood and well-being.

- *Touch grass (really):* Studies have shown that grounding, which is the practice of getting your bare hands or feet on natural surfaces, such as grass or soil, can lower stress hormones and reduce markers of chronic inflammation.

- *Additional strategies:* These are as individual as we are—find what works for you. Yoga, meditation, journaling, calling your bestie, exercising, setting boundaries, walking on the beach or hiking in nature . . . there are so many fantastic stress-reducing strategies.

- *Limit alcohol intake:* This may seem counterintuitive since it's common to reach for a drink to help us "relax," but our alcohol tolerance appears to plummet (we need more research on this) as our hormones do. Drinking can exacerbate feelings of anxiety and low mood during menopause, as well as dramatically disrupt our sleep.

SLEEP OPTIMIZATION

- Consider a wearable sleep tracking device—I use one, and it has helped me realize the habits that are affecting my sleep.

- Incorporate good sleep hygiene habits.

CHAPTER 10

The Menopause Tool Kit: A Symptom-Based Resource Section

My primary goal in creating this Tool Kit is to provide you with the tools that can help relieve menopausal symptoms and reduce associated increases in health risks. But I also want the Tool Kit to serve as a tool of expansion; I want it to open the minds of people (in the public and in the medical community) to the many ways menopause may manifest itself symptomatically.

I hope the lengthy list of potential symptoms will serve as validation that, yes, these symptoms exist outside of your experience, and yes, it's possible for them to arise as a result of hormonal changes that begin to happen during the menopausal transition. For far too long nonclassic symptoms of menopause have been dismissed by the medical community as solely a result of aging, and this dismissal has resulted in a failure to treat, validate, or evaluate patients needlessly suffering from menopausal symptoms.

If you've been dismissed or denied appropriate medical care and support in the past, I see you and I hear you and I am here for you. I hope that this Tool Kit empowers you to proactively manage your health and well-being during this significant life transition.

How to Use the Menopause Tool Kit

I think the Tool Kit will be mostly self-explanatory, but I do want to provide some notes that may be helpful. First off, you will find the entries listed in alphabetical order. Some symptoms have the same underlying cause and therefore a similar treatment approach, and I have grouped these together. For example, thinning hair, acne, body odor, and unwanted hair growth during menopause are all linked to a relative rise in androgens, so you will find suggested strategies listed under "Androgen-Induced Conditions" (and if you look up any of these problems, like body odor, singly, a cross-reference will direct you to the heading under which they are discussed).

You will notice that the number and type of strategies for each symptom vary. As I mentioned, this is because the research isn't as robust across the board for all symptoms. Some will have multiple approaches, including nutrition, pharmacology, supplementation, and exercise, while others may have only a pharmacological approach. In those that have strategies in multiple areas, my advice is to implement the nutrition strategy first, always, and then exercise, pharmacology, and supplements. Whichever strategy you decide to try, the key is to be consistent with it and be patient as you await noticeable improvement.

Acid Reflux/Gerd, see Gastrointestinal Issues

Acne, see Androgen-Induced Conditions

Androgen-Induced Conditions (Acne/Thinning Hair/ Body Odor/Unwanted Hair Growth)

Because these symptoms all have the same cause, I've included them in one entry.

During perimenopause, it's possible to see a *relative* increase in the production of androgens, the sex hormones such as testosterone that are typically associated with male characteristics like muscle development and facial hair growth. By *relative*, I mean that the rise in androgens isn't an isolated event but instead occurs as a response to other hormonal and chemical changes, including:

- LESS STEROID HORMONE BINDING GLOBULIN (SHBG). The decline in estrogen and progesterone production leads to the liver producing less steroid hormone binding globulin (SHBG). SHBG is a protein that binds to sex hormones while they travel in the bloodstream and renders them inactive, so when SHBG levels go down, there are more free and active androgens in the bloodstream.

- DECREASED CONVERSION OF ANDROGENS INTO ESTROGEN. Your number of ovarian follicles declines in perimenopause, and fewer follicles means less conversion of androgens into estrogen.

- CONTINUING ANDROGEN PRODUCTION BY THE ADRENAL GLANDS. Some androgens are produced by the adrenal glands, and their contribution becomes relatively more significant as ovarian estrogen production decreases. One trade-off is that the relative rise in androgens might lead to an increase in sexual desire for some women.

It's important to note that not all women experience a significant symptomatic rise in androgens during perimenopause, and the effects can vary widely among individuals. The balance of hormones during this transition is complex and influenced by genetic factors and overall health. In some individuals, the relative rise in androgens can lead to any of the four issues that follow.

Acne

I spent years battling changes that were happening in my body, not realizing that it was perimenopause. I didn't even know it was a thing! I was experiencing unexplained weight gain, cystic acne, depression, and erratic and highly irregular bleeding and I pursued various doctors, supplements, treatments . . . no one ever suggested that it could be perimenopause. My own ob-gyn—who is my age—commiserates with me but didn't have any answers—even for herself! It wasn't until I saw one of Dr. Haver's Facebook lives that it clicked for me! I ultimately had a hysterectomy as a result of the irregular bleeding, so I'm not sure where I am in my menopausal journey—unless I have a blood test to determine. In the meantime I am managing my symptoms by following the Galveston Diet. It has helped me reduce the frequency and severity of my symptoms and take control of my health in a way that no doctor had previously considered.

—Margaret W.

Acne is a chronic inflammatory disease that affects the hair follicle, hair shaft, and sebaceous gland units on your skin. If you had acne as a teenager or young adult, you are all too familiar with the many ways it may express itself, including as pore blockages, whiteheads, blackheads, and painful cystic pimples that may cause scarring.

Some people are surprised that acne can emerge or re-emerge during midlife, but it makes sense when you consider that acne is most likely to happen during times of hormonal upheaval, namely around puberty or perimenopause. This is because the sebaceous glands in your skin are controlled in large part by levels of androgens such as testosterone and DHEA; if you experience a relative increase in androgens during the menopausal transition, you may be at increased risk of developing adult-onset acne or, if you experienced it in adolescence, a recurrence.

We also become more prone to acne around menopause because of an increase in overall skin sensitivity caused by loss of moisture, collagen, and elastin. Sun exposure, cosmetics, smoking, medications, stress, and sleep loss can trigger acne in more sensitive, aging skin.

STRATEGIES FOR IMPROVING MENOPAUSAL ACNE

There are many options on the market for managing and improving adult acne, and the best treatment for you will vary based on the severity of your skin condition. Since treating acne can help minimize scarring, it's important not to delay.

Menopausal acne may be improved by being consistent with specific lifestyle habits, which on the plus side also happen to promote good overall health. These include taking steps to reduce stress; eating a low-sugar, high-fiber, antioxidant-rich diet; and exercising regularly. And if you have yet to incorporate a consistent skin care routine appropriate for midlife skin, please give yourself this gift. A pre-bed routine that promotes skin nourishment while you are sleeping is a must—and it can help reduce occurrences of acne.

If you have developed menopausal acne, consider seeing a dermatologist to help design a protocol that works best for the specifics of your skin condition. A protocol may include in-office procedures that can help treat acne scars and minimize skin aging.

Pharmacologic options: Mild acne can usually be treated successfully with prolonged topical therapy:

- TOPICAL RETINOIDS include prescriptions such as adapalene (0.3 percent), tretinoin, retinol, or retinaldehyde. Of these, tretinoin might be the most effective, but it can cause irritation in sensitive skin.

- BENZOYL PEROXIDE, available over the counter or by prescription, should be used with caution, as its use can lead to skin irritation and dryness.

- AZELAIC ACID is a prescription that has anti-inflammatory and antimicrobial properties. It can also help with postinflammatory hyperpigmentation.

- DAPSONE GEL is a prescription antimicrobial and anti-inflammatory treatment that is well tolerated and can be used as maintenance therapy for long periods.

- PRESCRIPTION COMBINATION THERAPIES with benzoyl peroxide and adapalene or tretinoin and clindamycin are effective as well but may have increased irritant potential.

- NONCOMEDOGENIC MOISTURIZERS may be used to reduce acne flare-ups.

Other options for treatment include the use of oral contraceptives, which can be helpful during perimenopause since they decrease the ovarian production of androgens. Sadly, MHT has not yet been studied as a treatment for menopausal acne.

If your acne is more moderate to severe or is resistant to topical treatment, a systemic therapy such as an antiandrogen or isotretinoin might be recommended. Spironolactone, a diuretic used in the treatment of high blood pressure, is commonly used off-label for its antiandrogen effect. It comes in pill form (prescription) and has proven helpful in improving hormonal and cystic acne.

Body Odor

> I had my progesterone IUD taken out when I was forty-three. My doctor told me I could still get pregnant but didn't mention hormone shock. My hair fell out (a lot), I started to see thinning around the crown of my head, I had a horrible onion body odor when I would sweat, and my lady parts also had something funky happening. I developed scalp acne, oily scalp, and dry skin all over. I did have more sex drive. My doctor told me that testing my hormones would be no help and told me nothing was wrong. I finally saw a naturopath who gave me herbs to adjust my progesterone levels, and discovered I was producing a lot of 5-DHT. I started taking saw palmetto and saw immediate improvement. After two years, I'm finally feeling myself. My hair is growing back, I don't smell, my lady parts aren't gross, and my oily scalp and dry skin are much better.
>
> —Nadine H.

The relative increase in testosterone during menopause can lead to higher concentrations of bacteria in sweat, which can alter body odor, and not for the better. Excessive perspiration during hot flashes and night sweats may also feed underarm bacteria, further intensifying odor. Increased stress and anxiety, common in menopause, can also modify the scent of your sweat (yes, stress really does stink).

STRATEGIES FOR MINIMIZING BODY ODOR

You can reduce body odor by getting control of hot flashes—and the excessive sweating they can cause—through the use of menopausal hormone therapy. This won't get rid of body odor entirely, but less sweat can lead to less stench.

Other approaches to body odor include the following:

- SAW PALMETTO is an oral herbal supplement derived from the fruit of a shrublike palm. Saw palmetto extracts have been shown to interfere with androgenic activity by blocking the conversion of testosterone to dihydrotestosterone (DHT), the androgen most associated with pungent body odor.

- SPIRONOLACTONE is a prescription that may help reduce body odor as well by blocking the effects of androgens on the skin. Talk to your doctor about prescribing this option.

- MANDELIC ACID applied to the skin can block bacteria's digestion of bodily fluids and is bacteriostatic and nonirritative. It is typically applied to the skin as a deodorant and is an alternative to the common deodorants that contain aluminum. My favorite brand is Lume Whole Body Deodorant.

Thinning Hair (on Head)

When I was in my late forties, I started experiencing many different symptoms—hip bursitis, knee pain, hair loss, sleep issues, urine leakage, breast tenderness, UTIs, frozen shoulder, skin rashes, and more. A few years before, I had been diagnosed with a thyroid disorder. At one point, I had an endocrinologist that was prescribing thyroid medication, I was seeing an orthopedic surgeon for the joint conditions, I was asking my gynecologist about the sexual dysfunction and breast tenderness, I was being treated by a urologist for the incontinence, and I was seeing a dermatologist for the hair loss and skin conditions. And the endocrinologist and the gynecologist argued about whether it was my thyroid or my female hormones that were still causing the lingering symptoms. Finally, I found an out-of-pocket endocrinologist in California that could help me with all of these symptoms. She started me on HRT, which solved many of my issues. She saw the hormonal system as one complete unit.

—Denise S.

Hair loss during menopause is common and often a cause of significant distress. It may occur as a response to many factors, including stress, medications, illness, and genetic predisposition, but it's primarily triggered by the relative increase in androgens that may begin to occur during the menopausal transition. There are a few ways hair loss typically may present itself in menopause:

- FEMALE PATTERN HAIR LOSS (FPHL) involves gradual hair thinning on the crown of the scalp, starting with thinning along the central hair part. The frontal hairline typically remains intact.

- TELOGEN EFFLUVIUM (TE), or sudden hair shedding, may arise after major life stressors, chronic illnesses, COVID, or specific medications that might lead to unintended hair loss. These two conditions can coexist, and FPHL might worsen following an acute TE episode.

- MALE PATTERN HAIR LOSS (MPHL), while less common, can occur in women and cause thinning or balding on the top of the head and recession along the temples.

- FRONTAL FIBROSING ALOPECIA (FFA), mainly seen in postmenopausal women, is an inflammatory condition that can lead to hair loss along the temples and overall hair loss, including in the eyebrows and eyelashes.

Other conditions, unrelated to menopause, including thyroid disease, cicatricial alopecias, trichotillomania, and alopecia areata, may also be potential causes of hair loss. It's important to consult a dermatologist to find out the root cause of your symptoms.

STRATEGIES FOR PREVENTING HAIR LOSS

With hair loss in menopause, the goal of treatment is typically to prevent further hair loss rather than to promote regrowth. For this reason, if you notice patterned hair loss developing and you're interested in preserving your hair, it's important to go to your dermatologist as soon as possible. Your doctor might also have you tested for any nutritional deficiencies, which can cause or worsen hair loss and may need to be corrected through supplementation.

Pharmacologic options: There are a handful of treatment options for hair loss available, but only one that's been FDA approved for the treatment of FPHL:

- TOPICAL MINOXIDIL (FDA-approved) promotes hair regrowth by prolonging the anagen phase and increasing follicle size, and it's commonly used alongside oral antiandrogens (such as spironolactone). I use minoxidil myself. I get the 5 percent men's extra strength and place it in a spray bottle, and I apply it three times a week in the evening onto my scalp in two-inch sections. Possible adverse effects include new and unwanted facial hair growth, contact dermatitis, and irritation. Minoxidil can initially cause increased hair shedding, aka "dread shed," but this will be followed by hair stabilization or improvement over four to six months.

Other treatments include:

- Low-level laser therapy

- Platelet-rich plasma therapy

- Hair transplantation

- Hormone treatments, antiandrogens, and estrogen therapy are also considered to be helpful, though there has yet to be conclusive evidence showing that MHT on its own is effective at promoting hair growth in postmenopausal women.

- Spironolactone is a prescription that competitively blocks androgens. This medication is FDA approved for the treatment of other conditions but not for hair loss. Still, it is often used by physicians as a treatment for hair loss.

- Finasteride, another prescription, is effective for male pattern hair loss but is not approved for women.

- Estrogen therapy and adjunctive therapies like bimatoprost, ketoconazole shampoo, and low-energy laser-light devices are also options.

- Camouflaging sprays, powders, and hairpieces can enhance the appearance of hair density.

Unwanted Hair Growth

Hirsutism is a condition in which women experience excessive, coarse, and/or dark hair growth in androgen-sensitive areas such as the chest, back, or face. The face, the chin, the upper lip, and the cheeks are the most androgen sensitive, so these are the areas where you're most likely to see increased hair growth.

The underlying cause of hirsutism always has something to do with androgens. During the reproductive years, unwanted hair growth can result when your ovaries overproduce androgens, which happens in polycystic ovary syndrome (PCOS), or when you have hypersensitivity to normal androgen levels (called idiopathic hirsutism). During menopause or your postreproductive years, you may experience unwanted hair growth due to an increase in androgens relative to the decrease in estrogens. (In a cruel twist of fate, you might inadvertently increase facial hair if you use minoxidil to treat female pattern hair loss.)

STRATEGIES FOR REDUCING UNWANTED HAIR GROWTH

Management of unwanted hair growth varies greatly depending on how frustrating or distressing it is to you. For some, a really good pair of tweezers and good lighting are all that they need. For others, this is not nearly enough "treatment." If you fall into this second group, you can see your dermatologist to get help devising a plan to target unwanted hair growth. The plan may include checking you for excess androgen levels and ruling out other abnormalities, then implementing treatment.

Pharmacologic options: Some treatment options include:

- Antiandrogen/androgen-blockers like spironolactone
- 5α-reductase inhibitors, such as finasteride and dutasteride
- Pharmacological therapy followed by mechanical hair removal, such as plucking, waxing, or shaving
- Bleaching and/or chemical depilatory agents
- Electrolysis or laser treatments (possible adverse effects include folliculitis, dyspigmentation, and tunneling of hair under the skin)
- Estrogen therapy may delay hirsutism progression but won't change coarse hairs into softer ones

Anxiety, see Mental Health Disorders and Mood Changes

Arthaligia; see Muskuloskeletal Pain

Arthritis; see Muskuloskeletal Pain

Asthma

Asthma is a condition where your airways become inflamed, leading to symptoms such as wheezing, coughing, or shortness of breath. While the inflammation that brings about symptoms is local to the lungs, systemic or chronic inflammation may play a role in the development or worsening of asthma.

Asthma is more common and severe in women when compared to men, a fact that has led to the belief that hormones and specifically estrogen may be a key factor involved. We know that in menopause the decrease in estrogen leads to less protection against inflammation throughout the body, leaving all body systems vulnerable to inflammatory diseases. This includes creating a susceptibility to disease or dysfunction in the lungs. Some studies have suggested that late-onset asthma, defined as asthma diagnosed after the age of forty, is triggered by the kind of systemic inflammation that may be introduced as estrogen levels fluctuate and decline. Unfortunately, late-onset asthma can be harder to treat than asthma that develops when you are younger, and it may be less responsive to anti-inflammatory medications.

Strategies for Addressing Asthma

Research has found that postmenopausal women with asthma have a more significant decrease in estrogen compared to postmenopausal women without asthma, suggesting that estrogen really does play a vital role in protecting respiratory health. For this reason, "replacing" estrogen is a key consideration when it comes to asthma in menopause, but so far the research has produced conflicting results. Let's take a look.

Research published in the medical journal *Asthma and Lower Airway Disease* found that hormone replacement therapy was associated with a reduced risk of development of late-onset asthma in menopausal women. Additional research determined that MHT was helpful in bringing estrogen levels back to normal in asthmatic women, and it was also shown to reduce symptoms related to menopause and asthma. However, there were conflicting results in another study published in 2021, which found that hormone therapy use was associated with the development of *new* asthma. In those who developed asthma, however, stopping MHT proved to be effective at eliminating their asthma.

I share all this information not to confuse you but to make sure you are getting the full picture. I suspect what's going on with respiratory health and MHT may be similar to what we've seen in the areas of cardiac or neurological health. That is, if an individual has a preexisting progression of inflammation in an area, hormone therapy may contribute to the inflammatory state rather than help correct it or ward off additional cellular damage. We've been able to use the timing hypothesis (see page 31) to help protect women who may be vulnerable to the progression of disease states in the heart and brain, but this hasn't been studied as it relates to the lungs. Until we have more conclusive science, I recommend discussing with your doctor the potential asthma-related symptoms to watch out for after starting menopausal hormone therapy. If new symptoms develop, you may need to consider decreasing or stopping MHT.

Autoimmune Disease (New or Worsening)

> Over the course of several years, I was diagnosed with one autoimmune disease after another—lichen sclerosus, frozen shoulder, rheumatoid arthritis, and IBD. They have all been diagnosed by either my GP or different specialists, thus no one was seeing the big picture. It was only after reading several menopause books which quickly mention autoimmune disease that I made the connection and approached my doctor. My periods had been heavy clots for over five years, then stopped. So we discussed that HRT made sense, and I have been using the estrogen patch and progesterone pills for one month now (I am fifty). Please dedicate some time to the link between autoimmune disorders and menopause!
>
> —Caroline L.

An autoimmune disease is characterized as the body's immune system attacking its own healthy cells and tissues. In a healthy immune response, inflammation is a good thing—it protects you from illness and helps you recover from injury—but too much of an inflammatory response can set the stage for autoimmunity to occur. There are over eighty autoimmune diseases, including rheumatoid arthritis, multiple sclerosis, Graves' disease and Hashimoto's (both diseases of the thyroid), and psoriasis. Women are twice as likely to have autoimmune disease, and they are most often diagnosed during times of profound stress or significant hormonal change. Menopause obviously checks both boxes!

The hormonal changes that happen during menopause have been found to affect inflammatory processes and cause disruptions in the function of your immune system, which is where autoimmune disease originates. The natural reduction in estrogen production also plays a part. As I've mentioned in earlier chapters, estrogen is profoundly anti-inflammatory and when it diminishes during the menopausal transition, a low-grade chronic proinflammatory state can be introduced.

Decreasing estrogen levels also seem to disrupt the ratio of neutrophils to lymphocytes, two key white blood cell types that play an important role in protecting you from viruses, bacteria, and disease. Researchers have found that during the menopausal transition, the ratio can get skewed and create an imbalance that increases the risk of autoimmune disease.

STRATEGIES FOR AUTOIMMUNE DISEASE

The following can be helpful in protecting against or relieving autoimmune disease:

- MENOPAUSAL HORMONE THERAPY (MHT) has been found to have a protective effect in individuals with rheumatoid arthritis, likely a result of estrogen's ability to potentially help reduce inflammation in your joints.

- VITAMIN D aids in regulation of the immune system and helps reduce inflammation, which is why it's not surprising that low levels of vitamin D have been identified as a key trigger in the development of autoimmune diseases. While there's no universal dosage, or amount of sunshine, that's been proven to prevent or improve autoimmune disease, supplementation has been shown to be beneficial. I recommend getting your vitamin D level checked annually and supplementing if your level falls below the recommended range.

- Research has shown that plant compounds called *flavonoids* may have an ability to protect against autoimmune disease by blocking the immune system from damaging itself. You can get flavonoids from foods such as apples, blueberries, onions, citrus fruits, and spinach, and from certain types of tea, including green tea.

- PROBIOTICS containing *Lactobacillus* and *Bifidobacterium* may help to promote a balance between immune cells, which is key to preventing autoimmune disease. Probiotics have also proven to be helpful in relieving gastrointestinal symptoms and reducing inflammation in rheumatoid arthritis, ulcerative colitis, and multiple sclerosis.

- CURCUMIN is a plant compound found in the golden yellow spice turmeric, and in supplements, and has been shown to have incredible healing properties. In the immune system, curcumin has an ability to counter the effects of cytokines, inflammatory proteins that contribute to the type of cellular damage present in autoimmune disease.

Bloating, see Gastrointestinal Issues

Body Composition Changes/Belly Fat

I thought I had the Golden Ticket: fifty-five years old, still getting my period like clockwork, and feeling like I am in my thirties—life was good! Until it wasn't (thank you, Covid, for drop-kicking me into full-blown menopause). Volcano eruptions of sweat started happening almost overnight! I was waking up three to four times during the night. I was wide awake, soaking wet, and wondering what the heck was happening to my body. On one of these sleepless nights, I rolled out of bed with sore shoulders, hips, and breasts, only to find my midsection protruding as if I was six months pregnant!! AND still, I heard from no one who had gone through this, and I thought to myself: Where are all my ladies that have journeyed through the lava, in silent pain? WHY? Why are we silently sitting in confusion? Shame? Disbelief? The thinking that we are somehow unique in this experience? Come on, ladies, this is real and serious, and we need to have the discussions and get healthy!

　　　　　　　　　　　　　　　　　　　　　　　　　　　　—Cyndi F.

Most of us have gained unwanted weight at some point during our lives; we know how it feels, how our bodies may change with this weight gain, and we have a few strategies we rely on to help us get back to where we want to be. And then there's the hormonal weight gain that can happen around perimenopause. It can feel sudden, more like a shape shift than a weight gain. It can be stubborn, not budging in response to those trusted strategies from before. It just feels *different*. Because it is.

As I mentioned in chapter 6, one of the main reasons people visit my office is this different, distinct, and often surprising sort of weight gain. I usually explain that there's a reason for it and that the reason is changing estrogen levels. As estrogen levels start to fluctuate in perimenopause and trend downward, changes in where we store fat can begin to occur, namely intraabdominal fat gain. You may start to feel as though your belly is pushing out, and your pants may begin to feel increasingly tight. This is likely happening because of the new deposition of visceral fat.

Visceral fat is a type of deep abdominal fat that can cause a lot of metabolic trouble by releasing inflammatory proteins, which have far-reaching effects. Visceral fat has been linked to high cholesterol, insulin resistance, and chronic inflammation, and is a risk factor for type 2 diabetes, cardiovascular disease, and cognitive impairment.

The problem is that estrogen loss seems to program us to gain visceral fat, with significant jumps seen in this type of fat between premenopause and postmenopause: One study showed that a premenopausal woman's total body fat is likely to be 5–8 percent visceral fat, whereas a postmenopausal woman's total body fat is 15–20 percent visceral fat.

The good news is that several strategies may help combat visceral fat gain. They may be different from what you've tried before, so I encourage you to keep an open mind!

Strategies for Dealing with Body Composition Changes

Many of the strategies mentioned in the general "Menopausal Best Practices" outlined earlier on page 144 will also work for addressing an increase in visceral fat. These include eating a diet that is high in natural fiber, lean protein, nuts, seeds, fruit, legumes, and antioxidants, and low in processed carbohydrates (I'll reiterate details in this entry for ease of use). A few strategies have been shown to specifically encourage and support belly fat loss, including:

- NOT SMOKING. If you smoke, stopping smoking can lead to significant changes in visceral fat loss and overall decreased risk of cardiovascular disease, stroke, and other metabolic disorders. (Visit the CDC, the American Cancer Society, or the American Lung Association websites for resources that can help you quit smoking.)

- FINDING THE RIGHT STRESS-REDUCTION PRACTICES FOR YOU. Stress increases levels of stress hormones such as cortisol that drive up inflammation and contribute to visceral fat gain. Plus, stress lowers quality of life and can only compound your experience of menopausal symptoms. During this time of our lives, it's imperative to prioritize finding the right stress-reducing practices. What worked in your twenties or thirties might not work now. Ask yourself: What brings me a sense of peace and calm? If your answers lead you to a practice, start doing more of whatever it may be. If you couldn't think of anything, here are a few ideas: taking short walks, getting more fresh air, journaling, using a meditation app, or engaging in sessions with a counselor or therapist.

- GETTING GOOD SLEEP. Studies have suggested that chronic sleep loss may be linked to increases in visceral fat. The challenge in menopause is finding ways to get quality sleep while dealing with disruptive night sweats and increases in other symptoms that can interfere with sleep, such as sleep apnea and anxiety. Revisit the Tool Kit entry on sleep disturbances for a list of strategies, but your first focus should be on improving your overall sleep hygiene. This means evaluating room temperature and bedding and clothing for comfort and eliminating possible noise or light disturbances.

I also encourage:

- ENGAGING WITH A COMMUNITY. You may feel entirely alone in dealing with the menopausal transition and its related symptoms, but countless others out there can relate to and understand what you're experiencing; connecting with them could help alleviate the sense of isolation you may be feeling. There's been an explosion of menopausal online communities in the last few years—they offer opportunities for connection and increased access to information. You can check out our community on the 'Pause Life website, Stripes, etc.

- TAKING A BASELINE MEASUREMENT. I've found that with a lot of my patients, determining their waist-to-hip ratio can be helpful in establishing a reliable marker by which you can measure any changes. To get your waist-to-hip ratio, measure your waist at the smallest point—usually at the navel or just above it—then measure your hips at the widest, largest part. Now divide your waist measurement by your hip measurement (waist measurement ÷ hip measurement). In women, a ratio of 0.85 or lower is an indicator that you are at a lower risk for developing certain diseases.

NUTRITION

Helpful nutritional strategies include:

- ADOPT AN ANTI-INFLAMMATORY DIET: A diet full of complex carbohydrates, lean proteins, and healthy fats (nuts, seeds, avocados, olive/avocado oils, fatty fish) will lower inflammation, support hormone production, and improve your overall health. Visit our website thepauselife.com for more information about *The Galveston Diet*.

- LIMIT ADDED SUGARS: Consume no more than 25 grams of added sugar per day. Added sugars are the sugars that are added in cooking and processing of foods and alcohol.

- INCREASE FIBER INTAKE: Aim to consume at least 25 grams of fiber per day. The majority of your fiber should come from food, but many struggle to reach this goal. I have created a fiber supplement for my patients and students; see thepauselife.com for details.

- EAT MORE PROTEIN: As I discussed on page 145, your specific protein needs may vary. But studies have shown that people who eat at least 1.2–1.6 grams of protein for every kilogram of ideal body weight have less belly fat, more muscle, and lower fragility scores (based on functional strength measures—grip strength, getting up off the floor, etc.) than people who eat less. Good sources of protein include whole eggs, fish, legumes, nuts, meat, and dairy products.

- GET PROBIOTICS FROM FOOD: Foods rich in probiotics include yogurt, sauerkraut, miso soup, soft cheeses, kefir, sourdough bread, acidophilus milk, and sour pickles. Consider a probiotic supplement if you are unable to get probiotics from food.

- CONSIDER INTERMITTENT FASTING (IF): Research has shown that IF may be an effective strategy to help reduce visceral fat. The PROFAST study demonstrated that twelve weeks of IF combined with a probiotic supplement in adults with obesity and prediabetes resulted in 5 percent body weight loss, lower blood sugar levels, and a significant reduction in total body fat, abdominal fat, and visceral fat and an increase in fat-free mass (muscle) as measured by DEXA. An additional study in 2022 found that IF combined with "paced protein" (protein-rich meals and snacks throughout the day) was superior to the standard caloric restriction diet in weight loss, body composition, cardiometabolic health, and hunger management. (There are several ways to intermittently fast, as I discuss at length in *The Galveston Diet*. What I recommend to my patients is to consider the 16:8 method of fasting, which instructs sixteen hours of continuous fasting and an eight-hour eating "window.")

EXERCISE

While you can't target visceral fat with abdominal exercises, getting consistent physical activity can introduce positive metabolic changes that promote visceral fat loss and prevent the gain of additional abdominal fat. Regular exercise is really going to be one of the most powerful "treatments" for helping correct hormone-driven body composition changes; one researcher went so far as to write that exercise is "critical in mitigating the accumulation of visceral fat during the menopause." A good balance of vigorous cardiovascular and strength training is going to deliver the metabolic benefits that promote a healthy waist-to-hip ratio, support bone and joint health, produce mood-boosting endorphins, and promote better sleep.

SUPPLEMENTATION

Some studies have shown that *omega-3 fish oil* and *fiber supplements* can help encourage visceral fat loss.

Probiotics have also been shown to help to specifically reduce belly fat with evidence revealing that *Lactobacillus*-based probiotics can reduce visceral and subcutaneous fat and *Bifidobacterium*-based probiotics can reduce visceral fat.

Borage oil has a high concentration of gamma-linoleic acid (GLA), a fatty acid that has been studied for its ability to reduce inflammation. In menopausal women, it's also been found to help promote a decrease in waist-to-hip ratio.

PHARMACOLOGIC OPTIONS

Research published in the *Journal of Clinical Endocrinology and Metabolism* noted that the use of menopausal hormone therapy (MHT) was associated with significant reductions in visceral fat. It's important to note, however, that this benefit was not seen in past users of hormone therapy, suggesting that if you plan to stop using HRT, it's important to have backup strategies in place.

The Hormones That Control Your Weight

Throughout this book, I've focused a lot on the complicated symphony of sex hormones, such as estrogen and testosterone, that takes place within your body and influences so much of what happens there. Well, there's another symphony taking place with what we might call your appetite hormones. These hormones play an important role in controlling hunger and creating the feeling of fullness (satiety), and they include insulin, leptin, ghrelin, cortisol, and a few key others. In *The Galveston Diet*, I covered these hormones extensively and created meal plans and recipes that could help optimize their function in menopause. If you haven't already, you can check out the book or online program at thepauselife .org for these resources, but you can also accomplish a great deal in the appetite hormone department by implementing many of the nutrition strategies addressed throughout the Tool Kit.

The use of GLP-1 agonist drugs like semaglutide is optional in the treatment of menopausal weight gain. As with any medication, the benefits must be weighed with the risks. My colleagues and I support the use of these medications if indicated, but caution to make sure the patient is consuming adequate protein intake and getting regular resistance training. These habits can help ensure that weight loss does not include excessive muscle loss, which creates an increased risk for osteoporosis and fracture.

Body Odor, see Androgen-Induced Conditions

Brain Fog

In the peak of perimenopause, I had constant brain fog. I couldn't focus and suffered in my work. My boss thought I was lazy, but he had no idea what I was going through. I worked out constantly and ate sensibly and saw no results; as a matter of fact, I gained weight primarily in my midsection and I appeared pregnant. I am now on my tenth week of HRT and I feel so much better. I'm still getting acclimated, but I do not have hot flashes at all and overall I feel a peace within me. I feel calm and no anxiety. I'm excited to see what the next few months will bring.

—Crystal B.

A noticeable change in brain function is common during the menopausal transition. This change is often described as "brain fog," although your doctor might be more likely to define it as cognitive decline or cognitive difficulty. Brain fog is most often related to alterations in learning and verbal memory and can manifest in difficulty in recalling names, words, or stories, and in an inability to maintain your train of thought or to recall why you walked into a room.

Brain fog is most likely to begin happening during perimenopause when your estrogen levels start to fluctuate. You have estrogen receptors in the hippocampus and prefrontal cortex, which are areas of the brain responsible for memory and other cognitive functions. When estrogen levels decline, these receptors may not be triggered to perform activities essential to recall, concentration, and focus, leaving you feeling about as sharp as a cotton ball.

Studies have shown that if you experience frequent hot flashes, you may be more likely to also experience memory difficulties, which can be made worse by mood issues and sleep disturbances (which may happen as a result of hot flashes . . . talk about a vicious cycle). The presence of menopausal symptoms may also indicate that your brain has undergone structural changes as a result of hormone shifts. The good news is that these changes appear to mostly reverse themselves over time.

Often menopausal brain fog creates feelings of concern because people fear it may be a sign of dementia. But dementia is rare before the age of sixty-four, so cognitive challenges that happen in your forties or fifties are more likely to be a result of declining hormone levels. Many if not most women will experience a reversal of memory difficulties once they become postmenopausal. (It's not like you'll reach menopause and then be handed the key to your memory back; it will be more like a gradual return to more familiar brain functioning.) However, some women with cognitive vulnerabilities, which can be introduced through genetic, environmental, or lifestyle factors, may be more susceptible to experiencing a continued decline of brain function.

Strategies for Minimizing Brain Fog

The loss of estrogen in menopause can have a big impact on your brain. Estrogen is neuroprotective, shielding brain cells from the effects of oxidative stress and amyloid beta toxicity, high levels of which have been linked to the type of cellular damage that occurs in Alzheimer's disease. Estrogen also appears to counteract the effect of stress hormones on the brain, furthering its offering of resilience and protection. As estrogen levels decline, we see brain function worsen in both cognition and mental health, perhaps a result of the multiple layers of protection lost. All of this is to say that the first line of defense in protecting the brain is most likely going to have something to do with returning estrogen to our bodies, but other strategies may also benefit brain function in menopause.

Generally, you can protect your long-term brain health and potentially reduce brain fog and risk for dementia by incorporating many of the same activities that will help create and maintain good overall health. These include:

- monitoring your blood pressure, cholesterol levels, and blood sugar and treating any high levels that are detected

- avoiding smoking or excessive drinking

- getting at least 150 minutes of moderate-intensity aerobic activity each week

- managing weight gain

- staying socially connected

- getting "cognitive exercise" regularly—reading, learning something new, or doing anything that might challenge your brain regularly

PHARMACOLOGIC OPTIONS

Some studies have shown that estrogen therapy may help restore protection against neuroinflammation and the effects of stress hormones on the brain. We need more research before we can confidently say whether hormone therapy improves memory and focus for all women during the menopausal transition. For now, the scientific insight has shown that:

- in individuals with menopause that occurred between the ages of forty and forty-five (early menopause), estrogen therapy may be helpful in maintaining cognitive function and lowering the risk of dementia.

- in other menopausal women, use of hormone therapy appears to be safe for cognitive function. But if your menopause occurred more than ten years ago, you'll want to pay special attention to the formulation you are using. Research has shown that in this group the use of conjugated equine estrogens (Premarin) and medroxyprogesterone acetate comes with increased risks, whereas oral estradiol plus progesterone has a neutral effect.

A lot of incredible work is being done to identify more evidence-based approaches for sustaining cognitive health as we move through menopausal hormone changes. Dr. Lisa Mosconi, who I first mentioned in chapter 4, discusses the most cutting-edge research in detail in her book *The Menopause Brain*; it's a must-read if you want to delve deeper into the neuroscience aspects of menopause.

NUTRITION

For added neuroprotection as you age, it's recommended that you make sure to get plenty of antioxidant micronutrients, such as vitamin C and vitamin E, and anti-inflammatory macronutrients, such as omega-3 polyunsaturated fatty acids.

- Some of the best dietary sources of vitamins C and E include sunflower seeds, almonds, leafy greens (beet greens, collard greens, spinach, and kale), citrus fruits, and cruciferous vegetables.

- For omega-3s, aim to consume cold-water fatty fish, such as salmon, mackerel, and sardines, and nuts and seeds, such as flaxseed, chia seeds, and walnuts.

Breast Tenderness/Soreness

My menopause story started when I was thirty-six. I went through a period of very tender and painful breasts. My right breast was so achy that I thought I had breast cancer. Thankfully, that went away but in my midforties it was replaced with insomnia, chronic dry eyes, and being hot at night. That eventually morphed into full-blown intense hot flashes, mostly at night. That stayed with me for two years. When I turned forty-nine, my doctor told me that my ovaries were done and I didn't have to worry about birth control anymore. The hot flashes went away—yay! I thought I was done; I was wrong! My hot flashes came back two years later and I'm still dealing with them. In March of this year, they went away. I hoped I was done. I was not because four weeks later, I started spotting, had nipple hardness, and was gassy/bloated, and the hot flashes returned . . . will this ever end? I'm beginning to have my doubts.

—Jennifer P.

Breast pain or tenderness, also known as mastalgia, commonly occurs in premenopause during your menstrual cycle or pregnancy, and it's reasonable to expect it to subside once those cycles stop. For some women, however, breast pain can stubbornly stick around and lead to fears that it may be a symptom of breast cancer. Breast pain, however, is rarely a symptom of breast cancer, regardless of age.

Breast pain can be either cyclical or noncyclical.

Cyclical breast pain is the most common type and is linked to menstruation. It is caused by monthly fluctuations of the hormones estrogen and progesterone, both of which have a stimulating effect on the breast tissue, causing it to retain water and increasing the size and number of ducts and milk glands.

If you are still menstruating, you may experience cyclical breast pain a few days before menstruation. Your breasts may become tender, painful, or lumpy, and the pain may extend to the upper and outer portions of the breast, the armpit, and the arm. Then, when menstruation ends, the symptoms usually subside. Cyclical pain may worsen during perimenopause, when hormones can surge and drop erratically, and linger into menopause, especially in women who use oral contraceptives or hormone therapy.

Noncyclical breast pain is not linked to menstruation and does not follow any predictable pattern. It may be constant or intermittent, affect one or both breasts, and involve the whole breast or just a small part. Noncyclical pain is usually a symptom of a specific problem, such as a cyst, a trauma, or a benign tumor. Several conditions affecting the chest wall, esophagus, neck and upper back, and even the heart can produce symptoms that are felt as breast pain.

If you have fibrocystic breast tissue, you could experience either cyclical or noncyclical pain in one or both breasts as a result. This very common condition can cause thickened tissue or an increased number of cysts in otherwise normal breasts and can lead to increased occurrence of pain, tenderness, or lumpiness.

You also may be more susceptible to breast pain if you have an imbalance in fatty acids within your cells, which may make your breast tissue more susceptible to hormonal changes.

Strategies for Dealing with Breast Pain

Breast pain may be relieved by wearing a supportive bra, avoiding caffeine and nicotine, and using ice packs or warm compresses. Evening primrose oil or fish oil supplements may also help alleviate symptoms.

Beyond these approaches, what works best for you will depend a great deal upon any underlying issues present. You may be advised to try:

- nonsteroidal anti-inflammatory drugs (NSAIDs)

- exercises for chest muscle strain or arthritis

- antibiotics for mastitis

- draining for an abscess or cyst

Brittle Nails

> Some days I feel frazzled for no apparent reason. In one second, I forget what I was told or what I was thinking. I feel like it's a pre-warning of dementia! The lack of quality and length of sleep is really taking a toll on me. I can fall asleep fast, but staying asleep is the issue. I am EXTREMELY tired all the time. Naps have become common. I've become a recluse. My skin is itchy, my nails are brittle, joints are achy, and my body has shifted fat around! I work out consistently but crave and consume SUGAR like it's the Holy Grail! I'm crankier (I swore I wouldn't be a grumpy old lady!). Bladder leakage during exercise is worse. Heart palpitations come out of nowhere, and some foods taste better/worse. Irregular periods! I WANT THIS OVER WITH!
>
> —Lorrie G.

Brittle nails are those that have become weak, dry, and/or more prone to breaking or splitting easily. Postmenopausal women are especially susceptible to weakened nails because of chemical changes that take place in the nails; our nail plates rely on a molecule called cholesterol sulfate for strength, and this molecule declines as we undergo hormone changes related to menopause.

You are also more likely to develop brittle nails if you have anemia or a thyroid disorder; wash your hands frequently; or are exposed to harsh chemicals regularly.

Strategies for Strengthening Brittle Nails

You can take good care of your nails by avoiding harsh chemicals and keeping them clean and dry. If you've developed brittle nails, additional strategies can be incorporated to help improve nail strength and condition.

Nutrition and supplementation strategies include the following:

- GET MORE BIOTIN, AKA VITAMIN B7. Biotin is a water-soluble vitamin that helps maintain healthy skin, hair, and nails. You can get it from foods such as eggs, nuts, and whole grains, and it's also available in supplement form.

- INCREASE TRACE ELEMENT INTAKE. Trace minerals are minerals that are required in small amounts for various physiological functions. Some trace elements in the form of supplementation that have been reported to be helpful for brittle nails include iron, zinc, and copper.

- ADD AMINO ACIDS. Your nails are largely composed of the protein keratin, and keratin is built by amino acids, especially cysteine. You can benefit nail health by eating cysteine-rich foods, such as poultry, eggs, beef, and whole grains.

As a pharmacologic option, estrogen therapy may also help. Because estrogen replacement therapy has a beneficial effect upon collagen, it may help improve the texture of your nails, but more studies are needed.

Burning Sensation in the Mouth/Tongue

> It all began for me after the birth of my third child. I was thirty-three years old and my periods became very sporadic. Initially, it was every three months, then every six months, until eventually by the time I was forty they had stopped altogether. My doctor ran all the tests. She put me on hormones to try and jump-start my periods. It didn't work. She performed a D&C due to thickening of the lining of my uterus. Ultimately, she concluded I was experiencing premature menopause. I then developed tingling and burning in my feet, and a burning tongue. My doctor sent me to a neurologist, who ran every blood test imaginable. I had biopsies on my legs to check my nerves and also in my arms. The blood tests all came back normal. The neurologist said my symptoms were idiopathic and essentially said, "Let me know if they get worse." No one ever suggested that it could possibly be menopause.
>
> —Patty V.

Burning mouth syndrome (BMS) is defined as experiencing a burning, tingling, scalding, tender, or numb sensation in the mouth despite there being no visible signs of injury. BMS is most commonly experienced on the tip of the tongue but is also felt in the lips, on the sides of the tongue, or on the roof of the mouth. Far more women than men experience BMS

(7:1 ratio), and the majority of patients with this frustrating and painful syndrome are middle-aged women who are postmenopausal.

We don't fully understand yet why menopausal women are more likely to deal with BMS, but one theory is that the dramatic fall of estrogen in and around menopause alters the production of chemical compounds that affect nerve function, and this disruption may be what causes pain and tingling in the network of nerves found in the mouth. Other researchers have suggested that our saliva may undergo changes that modify how the cells in our mouths perceive sensation.

Strategies for Alleviating Burning Mouth Sensation

The treatment options for BMS are intended to help improve symptoms, especially the symptom of pain, which can be disruptive and debilitating.

- The combination of a low-dose benzodiazepine, a tricyclic antidepressant, and gabapentin has shown to be effective in reducing pain.

- Topical or oral clonazepam can produce significant improvement in pain ("topical" in this case means sucking on a clonazepam pill more like a lozenge to get the most significant effects of the medication locally, i.e., in the mouth).

- It might sound strange, but diluted hot pepper sauce can also reduce oral pain associated with BMS (and yes—they actually did a research study to test this). Hot pepper sauce contains capsaicin, which can produce relief by desensitizing oral tissue. Try applying a 1:2 hot sauce to water ratio to the areas of your mouth most affected three to four times a day.

- Previous studies have looked at whether MHT is effective at reducing symptoms of BMS, and the results have been mixed. It might be helpful and could be worth a try, especially if you are already considering taking hormone therapy for other reasons.

- In research studies, some patients with BMS found the antioxidant alpha-lipoic acid produced significant improvements in symptoms, while others found it to be ineffective. Despite the mixed results, if you are looking for a non-prescription-based option to try, alpha-lipoic acid is available in supplement form and could work for you.

- You may hear that St. John's wort can help with burning mouth symptoms, but researchers who investigated its use found it did not produce a significant reduction in pain.

Chronic Fatigue Syndrome, see Fatigue

Crawling Skin Sensations/Tingling Extremities/ Electric Shock Sensations

> My hot flashes brought pain with them. I started peri at forty-seven and started having consistent flashes every forty minutes, day and night, and they hurt . . . like surface nerve pain all over my body. My blankets and even my clothes aggravated the pain. Doctors told me either they never heard of anything like it or the two were unrelated. In either case nothing could be done. Finally, at sixty-two to sixty-three, the pain subsided, and the flashes slowed down. I'm almost sixty-five now and I'm down to three to five flashes a day and no more pain. I've been to several doctors with no offer of MHT. But then I don't live in an area that promotes or supports it. I feel better now, but skin, hair, facial hair, and weight gain still plague me.
>
> —Angela P.

Dysesthesias and *paresthesias* refer to abnormal sensations experienced in the skin, such as electric shocks, tingling, crawling feelings, or burning sensations. These are forms of peripheral neuropathies that result from problems in the peripheral nervous system, which includes nerves outside the brain and spinal cord. Peripheral neuropathies can have various causes, including underlying medical conditions, injuries, and, as recent research suggests, hormonal changes associated with menopause.

A lot of the research is finding that the potential link between dysesthesias and paresthesias is particularly relevant in postmenopausal women. Estrogen contributes to nerve protection and regeneration, which is why a decline in estrogen levels may lead to peripheral neuropathy and create changes in pain sensitivity. And it seems like the more time away from estrogen, the more likely you are to develop this condition.

Strategies for Dealing with Crawling Skin Sensations/ Tingling Extremities/Electric Shock Sensations

If you do develop any of these sensations, it's important to see your doctor, as there are multiple potential causes; they may be endocrinologic in origin or a result of an autoimmune condition, a nutritional deficiency, a herniated disc, or some other cause that needs to be treated. The best treatment approach will depend on the underlying cause.

While the link between hormonal changes and peripheral neuropathy is becoming clearer, the role of menopausal hormone therapy (MHT) in alleviating these symptoms remains a subject of research.

Decreased Desire for Sex, see Sexual Dysfunction

Dental Problems

> My first symptom of menopause was weight gain, then came fatigue and the gum/teeth problems. Don't forget to mention the gum and teeth problems! I saw doctors and dentists. All told me I was losing my mind.
>
> —Kelly C.

Believe it or not, your dentist might be the first person to identify changes in your body related to menopause. This is because hormonal changes can alter your overall oral health and negatively affect your teeth and gums in several surprising ways. During perimenopause and post-menopause, you are at increased risk of:

- more plaque buildup

- gingivitis or advanced periodontitis

- dry mouth (noticeable if your lips start sticking to your teeth or your tongue feels dry to the touch)

- tooth sensitivity, pain, or decay

- deterioration of bone in your jaw, which can result in tooth loss and receding gums

- reduced saliva production

- bleeding or irritated gums

Strategies for Addressing Dental Problems

It's crucial that you develop a daily (or really twice-daily) dedication to good oral hygiene habits to help prevent or improve dental issues that may arise around menopause. Good oral hygiene includes:

- brushing your teeth twice a day and making sure to get your gumline and hard-to-reach areas

- flossing at least once a day

- getting regular checkups at your dentist and communicating any changes in your oral health that you've noticed

You can also support the health of your teeth, gums, and mouth by:

- eating an anti-inflammatory diet that includes plenty of leafy greens, cruciferous vegetables, olive oil, avocado, cold-water fatty fish, and berries

- limiting your intake of caffeine, alcohol, and high-sugar and high-salt foods

- staying hydrated

Implementing practices that reduce stress can benefit oral health too. When we are anxious or stressed, we are more likely to grind our teeth, which can cause oral irritation, and our immune system may become compromised, leaving us vulnerable to fever blisters (if you've had prior exposure to the herpes simplex virus-1) or mouth ulcers, aka canker sores. Pick a favorite stress-reduction technique and make a commitment to practice it daily if possible.

PHARMACOLOGY OPTIONS

There's promising research that shows hormone therapy may support oral health and help alleviate oral symptoms that can arise around menopause. One study found that around two-thirds of menopausal women with oral symptoms experienced relief after hormone replacement therapy. This isn't surprising when you consider that general oral discomfort is far more likely to be reported in perimenopausal and postmenopausal women than in premenopausal women, a fact that tells us hormone changes are involved in disrupting oral health (and hormone replacement might help).

Depression, see Mental Health Disorders and Mood Changes

Difficulty Concentrating, see Brain Fog

Dizzy Spells, see Vertigo

Dry or Itchy Eyes

Menopause was not kind to me! My hot flashes were so bad, some days I didn't leave the house. I remember reading the newspaper (fourteen years ago) and sweat dripping off my forehead onto the paper and dripping down my back. My dry eye symptoms started then, and I just thought I had an infection when I would have a flare-up with redness in my eye or eyes. I threw all my eye makeup out twice before I realized what it was. My hair was like straw and my skin became dry and lax. When I saw myself in store mirrors I almost didn't recognize me. Every joint in my body ached, even my toes. The fatigue was terrible. I was finally diagnosed with Hashimoto's and meds helped. I was too scared of hormone therapy then. My advice now to anyone who will listen is [to consider] HT.

—Jacki D.

Dry eye disease (DED) is a common eye condition that affects the surface of the eye. It can cause discomfort, pain, and changes in vision, and can generally disrupt your ability to focus and function as you move through your daily life. This condition is prevalent in women, especially those who are peri- or postmenopausal.

While a lot of factors can cause DED, decreasing hormone levels may on their own bring on dry eye disease. This is because the balance of estrogens and androgens plays an important role in the production of tears and the maintenance of the watery layer that moisturizes and protects the surface of your eyes. When this layer is disrupted, you are more prone to developing DED.

Strategies for Improving Dry Eye Disease

You can improve symptoms of DED with lifestyle changes, strategic supplementation, and medication use as needed.

According to the National Eye Institute, the most effective lifestyle strategies to help preserve eye health and relieve symptoms of dry eye disease include:

- avoiding smoke, wind, and excessive air conditioning

- adding moisture to dry indoor environments with a humidifier

- taking breaks from electronic devices to reduce eye strain, and limiting screen time when possible

- wearing wraparound sunglasses when outdoors

- staying hydrated by drinking enough water daily

- getting seven to eight hours of sleep per night

SUPPLEMENTATION

Several vitamins are crucial to maintaining the protective layer on your eyes, and deficiencies in some of these, specifically vitamins D, A, and B, can put you at an increased risk of developing DED.

- omega-3 fatty acids: at least 1,000 mg/day

- vitamin A: 5,000 IU/day

- vitamin D: no established dosage, but not to exceed 4,000 IU/day unless supervised by a physician

- vitamin E: 400 IU/day

PHARMACOLOGIC OPTIONS

Hormone replacement therapy has been suggested as a potential treatment for menopause-associated dry eye symptoms. Discussing MHT options with a healthcare provider can help women manage hormonal imbalances and alleviate DED symptoms.

For those who prefer non-MHT approaches or want to use them as complementary treatments, several other options are available:

- OVER-THE-COUNTER EYE DROPS: Mild DED can often be managed with artificial tears, which are readily available without a prescription. These eye drops can provide relief from dryness and discomfort.

- PRESCRIPTION MEDICATIONS: In more severe cases, prescription medications like cyclosporine (Restasis) or lifitegrast (Xiidra) may be recommended by an eye doctor. These medications can help the eyes produce more tears and reduce inflammation.

Dry Mouth, see Dental Problems

Dry Skin, see Skin Changes

Eczema, see Skin Changes

Electric Shock Sensations, see Crawling Skin Sensations

Fatigue

I thought I had long COVID or something seriously wrong with me. I had palpitations, anxiety, tinnitus, fatigue, insomnia, depression, and mood swings. I had stopped working out because I thought I had heart issues, and this only made my symptoms worse. I was checked out by a cardiologist and put on a low-dose beta-blocker (my BP was high), but that was it. I saw my primary doctor and he ran tests. My cholesterol was high. He wanted to give me a pill for each symptom: a statin, antidepressant, a sleeping pill, etc. Then I found Dr. Haver's social media account and I made an appointment with my gynecologist. I gave him a list of my issues, we discussed HRT, and I started taking estradiol and progesterone. BAM! I got my life back! I am back to the gym and now working on my nutrition.

—Cindy S.

With busy lives and multiple pulls on our energy as we age and gain responsibilities, being tired is too often the norm. But the kind of fatigue that can occur during menopause is more than just feeling tired after a long day—it can be physically and mentally exhausting and create an almost unbearable sense of heaviness or need to lie down. I find this is one of the key factors chipping away at the resilience of my patients over time.

Studies also show that fatigue is a very common symptom during perimenopause and postmenopause. In one cross-sectional study of three hundred women, increasing feelings of fatigue were associated with progressing through the menopausal stages. The study revealed that:

- 19.7 percent of premenopausal women reported symptoms of physical and mental exhaustion

- in perimenopause, there was a jump to 46.5 percent

- in postmenopause, an alarming 85.3 percent of women experienced fatigue

The question is: Why does this happen? The answer can be found in the hormonal changes that accompany menopause. As your body adjusts to the reduction in estrogen and progesterone production, other hormones, like those from the adrenal and thyroid glands, can behave differently. These hormones regulate energy usage in the body, and any imbalance can lead to feelings of tiredness.

And then there's the additional tiredness that results from menopausal symptoms like hot flashes and night sweats, which can cause frequent awakenings during the night and trouble falling back asleep, all of which can disrupt sleep patterns and promote daytime fatigue even more.

Increased fatigue during menopause can also be exacerbated by other factors that may develop during this time of your life. These factors include:

- SLEEP APNEA: Sleep disorders like sleep apnea are more likely to develop as we age and can lead to poor sleep quality and daytime fatigue. It's essential to rule out such conditions with a healthcare provider.

- MEDICATIONS: Some prescription medications—especially those that may help treat anxiety or depression—can have side effects such as fatigue.

Strategies for Reducing Fatigue

SLEEP

This sounds obvious, but it's important to say it anyway: If you're experiencing menopause-related fatigue, it's all the more important that you guard your sleep. One of the most effective strategies for getting more sleep is creating the ideal sleep environment. This includes setting the right temperature (between 60 and 67 degrees) in your bedroom and creating a comfortable sleep environment—remove any bright lights or disruptive noises, wear lightweight clothing, and make sure your bedding is appropriate to the room temperature. It's also recommended that you eliminate your exposure to blue light–emitting devices (cellphone, tablet, LED TV screens) two or more hours prior to bedtime.

EXERCISE

When you are feeling fatigued, the very thought of exercise can be a non-starter and make you feel even more exhausted. But we know that exercise can improve sleep quality (which in turn will help your fatigue levels) as well as boost your energy levels. While there haven't been a lot of studies looking at specific types of exercise and fatigue in postmenopausal women, one 2023 study did find that study participants who completed three thirty-minute Pilates workouts each week for eight weeks reported reduced general, physical, and mental fatigue. What this means is simple: Anything you can do to move your body on a regular basis will only reduce your level of exhaustion.

PHARMACOLOGIC OPTIONS

Because it helps stabilize hormone fluctuations that underlie the common and debilitating symptom, menopausal hormone therapy may help reduce your fatigue.

Chronic Fatigue Syndrome

Chronic fatigue syndrome (CFS), also known as myalgic encephalomyelitis (ME), is a complex and often debilitating condition characterized by persistent and unexplained fatigue, as well as a range of other symptoms such as pain, cognitive impairment, and sleep disturbances. There is ongoing research exploring the connection between CFS and menopause. A definitive link has yet to be established, but there have been a lot of important observations, including:

- *CFS predominantly affects women.* Interestingly, the majority of CFS cases are diagnosed during the reproductive years, as well as before or around the time of menopause. The fact that these periods in a woman's life are all hormonally charged and the gender disparity in CFS raise questions about hormonal influences, including those related to menopause.

- *Hormonal fluctuations may contribute to the development of or exacerbation of CFS symptoms.* Low-grade inflammation is considered to be a significant factor in the onset of chronic fatigue syndrome. Given what we know about estrogen's role in helping regulate the immune system and in keeping inflammation down, the loss of estrogen during menopause may contribute to the development or exacerbation of CFS symptoms.

- *Gynecologic surgeries may be linked to CFS.* Women who have undergone hysterectomy (removal of the uterus) and oophorectomy (removal of one or both ovaries), especially if they result in early menopause, may be at an increased risk of experiencing CFS symptoms.

- *Menopause can aggravate symptoms.* Some women report a worsening of CFS symptoms during perimenopause and menopause. The associated hormonal changes can lead to increased fatigue, sleep disturbances, and mood fluctuations, which may also interact with existing symptoms of CFS.

- *Overlap of symptoms.* Chronic fatigue syndrome shares some symptoms with menopause, including fatigue, sleep disturbances, and mood changes. This overlap in symptoms can make it challenging to distinguish between the two conditions, potentially leading to misdiagnosis or delayed diagnosis.

As research continues to focus on gaining a greater understanding of chronic fatigue syndrome and its origins, we may find that hormonal changes play an even bigger role than suspected. Hopefully, future insights will provide improved treatments for this complicated and disabling illness.

Fatty Liver Disease, see Nonalcoholic Fatty Liver Disease

Fibromyalgia, see Musculoskeletal Pain

Frozen Shoulder

Frozen shoulder, medically known as adhesive capsulitis, is characterized by stiffness and pain in the shoulder joint. This complex and poorly understood condition typically progresses through three stages: the painful phase, the frozen phase, and the thawing phase. During the painful phase, patients experience increasing shoulder pain, especially at night, which is often severe and disrupts sleep. The frozen phase is characterized by a gradual loss of range of motion, while the thawing phase involves the slow recovery of shoulder function over time. The causes of frozen shoulders can vary, including injury, inflammation, and underlying medical conditions.

Emerging research is showing that the loss of estrogen in menopause may be linked to incidence of frozen shoulder. This wouldn't be surprising since we know that estrogen plays a crucial role in stimulating bone growth, reducing inflammation, and maintaining the integrity of connective tissues; changes in any of these areas could set the stage for a condition such as frozen shoulder to develop.

In 2022, when researchers from Duke University looked into the potential connection between postmenopausal women, hormone replacement therapy (MHT), and frozen shoulder, they found some groundbreaking insights. The researchers looked at medical records from nearly two thousand postmenopausal women aged forty-five to sixty, all of whom presented with shoulder pain, stiffness, and adhesive capsulitis. They made some fascinating findings, including the fact that estrogen replacement therapy appeared to potentially help prevent frozen shoulder. In this study, women who took hormone replacement therapy (MHT) had a lower percentage (3.95 percent) of cases of frozen shoulder compared to women who didn't (7.65 percent). Although the differences in the numbers weren't big enough to be sure they weren't due to chance, they do make us wonder whether estrogen might have a role in preventing frozen shoulder. The researchers from Duke University felt confident that the drop in estrogen during menopause could be linked to the development of frozen shoulder. Before this study, the potential origins of frozen shoulder in menopausal women were poorly understood, which is why even the suggestion of a link to menopause was considered groundbreaking. At least now we have a starting point around which additional research can be built and potential treatments can be designed. While further research is warranted to establish a more concrete hormonal connection, we can hope that there is soon more evidence on how to best prevent and treat this painful condition.

Strategies for Dealing with Frozen Shoulder

The cornerstone of frozen shoulder treatment is physical therapy, and the sooner you get treatment the better, as this will help prevent further stiffness and loss of function. A physical therapist will help you gradually regain shoulder mobility through exercises, stretches, and manual techniques. They also might encourage the use of heat and ice to help lessen pain and reduce inflammation.

Pharmacological options include:

- MEDICATIONS: In the painful phase of frozen shoulder, nonsteroidal anti-inflammatory drugs (NSAIDs) and pain relievers can help manage discomfort and inflammation. These medications are typically prescribed to alleviate the severe pain associated with the condition. However, their long-term use should be monitored by a healthcare professional.

- CORTICOSTEROID INJECTIONS: In some cases, corticosteroid injections into the shoulder joint may be recommended to reduce inflammation and relieve pain. These injections can provide short-term relief, but their efficacy in the long run is limited. They are often used as part of a broader treatment plan in conjunction with other therapies.

Medical procedures include:

- HYDRODILATATION: Hydrodilatation is a procedure in which the shoulder joint is injected with sterile water to expand the joint capsule. This can help break up adhesions and increase the range of motion. It is often performed under ultrasound guidance and may be combined with corticosteroid injections.

- MANIPULATION UNDER ANESTHESIA (MUA): For people with severe frozen shoulder that does not respond to other treatments, MUA may be an option. This is a procedure where the patient is placed under anesthesia and the shoulder is manipulated to break up adhesions and improve mobility. It is typically followed by an aggressive rehabilitation program.

- SURGICAL INTERVENTION: Surgery is rarely considered for frozen shoulder, but it may be an option when all other treatments have failed. Surgery involves releasing the joint capsule to improve range of motion. Postoperative physical therapy is essential to achieve the best outcomes.

Gastrointestinal Issues

Prior to menopause I was petite: 5' 3" and 110 pounds after three children. I did moderate exercise, could eat absolutely anything and not gain weight, slept well, and had a lot of energy. Menopause hit, and then like a light switch, I went from feeling full of life and energy to no energy, stressed, angry, and no sleep. I could not explain the constant achiness and why I felt bloated all the time. I suddenly had a tire in my midsection, and there was nothing I could do to get rid of the bloating and excess weight gain. I gained thirty pounds in two years and honestly did not feel that I had changed any eating or exercise patterns. Then I had a consultation with my doctor who specialized in menopause, and after starting hormone therapy and understanding my diet a little bit better, coupled with intermittent fasting, I have lost some weight, but inches just dropped everywhere. I went down a size in my clothes, but mostly my quality of life is so much better and improving daily!

—Donna M.

The human gastrointestinal (GI) tract is a complex system responsible for the digestion, absorption of nutrients, and elimination of waste products. Recent research has found that estrogen and its receptors play a vital role in maintaining the health and functionality of this intricate system. When estrogen is depleted in menopause, its absence can influence gastrointestinal disease and discomfort, potentially contributing to the development of several conditions.

Acid Reflux/GERD (Gastroesophageal Reflux Disease)

When you have GERD, stomach acid flows backward into the esophagus, which can lead to heartburn, a feeling as if you have a lump in your throat, and trouble swallowing. Until age fifty, men are more likely to have GERD than women, but after menopause this increases dramatically for women. In fact, research has found that postmenopausal women were *3.5 times more likely to have GERD* when compared with premenopausal women. Estrogen might help delay the onset of acid reflux (GERD) by reducing inflammation and making the lining of the esophagus more resistant to the stomach acid that causes GERD.

Interestingly, women who have never used postmenopausal hormone therapies have a lower risk of reflux symptoms compared to those who have taken or are still taking estrogen replacement therapy. And risk of reflux symptoms increases with higher estrogen doses and longer durations of estrogen use. Selective estrogen receptor modulators (SERMs) and over-the-counter hormone preparations have also been associated with increased GERD risk.

What this tells us is that the lower esophageal sphincter may be especially responsive to estrogen replacement, becoming too relaxed and therefore *increasing* the risk of GERD among those taking hormone therapy or using therapies that promote estrogen production during menopause. GERD is one the few menopause-related symptoms that doesn't seem to get better after MHT. Some experts believe that this could be a side effect of *oral* estrogens only and that nonoral methods could have no effect on disease, but . . . we need more studies.

Irritable Bowel Syndrome (IBS)

IBS is a fairly common GI disorder affecting the large intestine and causing symptoms like abdominal pain, bloating, and altered bowel habits, such as an increase in constipation and/or diarrhea. Sex hormones, especially estrogen, play a big role in how our digestive system works and how it can go wrong. IBS is more common in women than men, and its symptoms can change during different parts of a woman's menstrual cycle, during pregnancy, and of course, after menopause. So researchers have linked sex hormones and gastrointestinal function, but there's still a lot we don't know about the interplay between the two. Research has shown that estrogen affects the motility of the colon, potentially contributing to IBS symptoms. After menopause, women with IBS tend to experience more severe IBS symptoms compared to women who haven't gone through menopause yet. However, this age-related change isn't observed in men with IBS. This difference is likely because female sex hormones have a strong influence on how the brain and gut communicate, affecting how women perceive stomach discomfort and how their digestive system works.

Colon Cancer

Colon cancer is a malignant tumor affecting the GI tract and is a leading cause of cancer-related mortality worldwide. Interestingly, females have a higher prevalence of colon cancer than males. Remarkably, the Women's Health Initiative study demonstrated a 30 percent reduction in the prevalence of colon cancer following MHT treatment in postmenopausal women. This suggests a potential protective role of estrogen in colon cancer.

Changes to the Gut Microbiome

Gastrointestinal issues during menopause can also be brought on by changes to the gut microbiome. The gut microbiome is the complex community of microorganisms residing in the digestive tract that plays a pivotal role in maintaining our overall health. This vital gut community is influenced by several factors, including aging and sex hormones, and research is starting to reveal the complex relationship between menopause and the gut microbiome. Menopause has been linked to the following microbiome changes:

- REDUCED MICROBIAL DIVERSITY: Menopause and lower estrogen levels have been associated with a decrease in the diversity of the gut microbiome. This decrease can disrupt the delicate balance within the microbiota, potentially leading to health complications.

- SHIFT TOWARD MALE-LIKE COMPOSITION: Research suggests that menopause may alter the gut microbiome composition, shifting it to be more like the male microbiome. While we don't know yet how this may correlate to changes in health, menopause-related microbiome alterations have been linked to adverse cardiometabolic profiles, which may include high blood sugar, high cholesterol, and increased waist circumference.

- ESTROBOLOME POTENTIAL: A new area of research is related to the estrobolome, which is a collection of enzyme-producing genes found in the gut microbiome that allow your gut bacteria to metabolize estrogen. Interestingly, the actions of the estrobolome allow for inactive estrogen to become active again and re-enter the bloodstream. During menopause, there may be a reduction in estrobolome potential, which could affect estrogen metabolism and hormone-related health. Researchers are exploring the potential role of the estrobolome as it relates to estrogen-responsive cancers, and I suspect we'll be hearing a lot more about it in the future.

- INCREASED GUT BARRIER PERMEABILITY: The decline in estrogen and progesterone levels during menopause may lead to increased permeability of the gut barrier. Greater permeability can allow bacteria and their by-products to cross into the bloodstream and potentially trigger inflammation.

Strategies for Mitigating Gastrointestinal Issues

I suspect future science will continue to reveal an increasingly meaningful connection between menopause and the gut microbiome and the ways this connection affects gastrointestinal health. We will also hopefully have more evidence-based strategies to offer in the years to come. For now, here are some strategies that can support your gut microbiome and gastrointestinal health.

NUTRITION

Eating a fiber-rich diet is the most important nutritional strategy for gut health. Fiber serves as a source of nourishment for beneficial gut bacteria, promoting their growth and the production of short-chain fatty acids, which benefit gut health. Fiber can also support digestion and minimize pressure on the lower esophageal sphincter, which can reduce heartburn and other symptoms of GERD. Ideally, women should get a minimum of 25 grams of fiber per day in their food—but most are only getting half that amount.

Some of my favorite sources of fiber include avocado (my favorite), beans, broccoli, berries, and chia seeds (see page 145 for expanded list). Fiber supplements can be helpful as well, but the majority of your fiber should come from food sources. See page 145 for a discussion on fiber supplements.

SUPPLEMENTATION

Foods rich in probiotics (yogurt, kefir, sauerkraut, etc.) and probiotic supplements containing strains like *Lactobacillus* species *casei, helveticus, rhamnosus,* and *reuteri* have shown promise in supporting postmenopausal gut health, which can in turn protect you from health risks that increase as hormone levels diminish. These probiotics can influence intestinal calcium absorption, reduce bone density loss, improve genitourinary symptoms, promote vaginal pH balance, and help manage cardiometabolic risk factors.

The Potential of Probiotics

Probiotics are nonharmful bacteria found in foods and supplements that may promote the growth of "good" bacteria in the gut. These so-called good bacteria can have a positive impact on your health by increasing absorption of nutrients, fighting off infection and other disease-causing elements, contributing to the prevention of food intolerance and allergy, and much more. Because a great deal of your health starts in the gut microbiome, you may notice that probiotics pop up as a strategy for many different symptoms of menopause. While there is limited evidence on the precise impact of probiotics (it can be difficult to isolate their effect), there is a lot of research demonstrating their significant potential in supporting your health—especially as you enter menopause.

For a 2023 article published in *Current Nutrition Reports,* researchers reviewed several randomized trials on the use of probiotics in menopause and found that probiotics may have a "pleiotropic effect," meaning that they could benefit various functions and systems. They may benefit health in menopause by:

- increasing calcium absorption, which may protect bone density and delay bone damage associated with the loss of estrogen in menopause

- reducing vaginal pH, which may protect against endometrial hyperplasia by limiting the activity of pathogenic bacteria

- protecting against inflammation, elevated cholesterol levels, and insulin resistance, which can collectively reduce your risk for metabolic syndrome and cardiovascular disease

- reducing incidence of breast cancer—likely related to the probiotics' effect on estrogen metabolism in the estrobolome—and improving genitourinary symptoms that can result from breast cancer therapy

It's important to note that for women in the study, probiotics that contain *Bifidobacterium* and *Lactobacillus* species *casei, helveticus, rhamnosus,* and *reuteri* seemed to have the most positive effect.

Genitourinary Syndrome

The genitourinary system includes our genital and urinary organs. In menopause, when we develop symptoms that affect the vagina, vulva, and/ or bladder, doctors refer to it as genitourinary syndrome of menopause (GSM). GSM has a wide range of symptoms and, despite being very common, often goes untreated because women *don't report symptoms out of embarrassment or lack of awareness* about the many effective treatment options. Let's look at specific organs and the various changes that can be brought on by estrogen loss in menopause.

In the bladder, supportive tissues in the region can weaken, leading to urinary incontinence. And the lining of the bladder and urethra become more susceptible to irritation and infection. Estrogen deprivation is the most likely cause of chronic UTIs in the menopausal woman.

In the clitoris, less blood flow and diminished tissue health reduce clitoral sensitivity and responsiveness. Less sensitivity and responsiveness in the clitoris often lead to decreased sexual arousal and pleasure.

In the vulva (opening of and external parts of the vagina, including the labia), the skin and mucous membranes can become thinner and lose elasticity. You can also experience decreased lubrication. The combined effect of these changes may result in irritation, discomfort, and dryness in the vulva, which may be most noticeable during sexual activity.

In the vagina, tissue can become thinner and lose elasticity, and vaginal lubrication can lessen. This can cause vaginal burning, itching, dryness, and pain during intercourse. You may also become more susceptible to vaginal infections.

Strategies for Dealing with Genitourinary Syndrome

Symptoms of GSM can significantly affect a woman's quality of life and intimate relationships. The good news is that you don't have to endure these symptoms because there are many treatment options that can produce relief and reintroduce sexual pleasure, if that's a goal. Because GSM symptoms can also be caused by infection, it's important to see your gynecologist as soon as possible if you are experiencing any of the possible symptoms mentioned. When you get to your appointment, be honest and open about your symptoms so that you ensure you get the most effective treatment available. That said, the most effective long-term treatment for the prevention of UTIs in a menopausal woman is vaginal estrogen, not antibiotics.

Pharmacologic options include:

- VAGINAL ESTROGEN: Low-dose vaginal estrogen therapy is considered the gold standard for treating GSM. It is safe, cost-effective, and effective for most women with this condition. It is available in a pill, gel, or ring form. See chapter 7 for a full discussion on vaginal estrogen therapeutic options.

- INTRAVAGINAL DEHYDROEPIANDROSTERONE (DHEA): DHEA, applied usually in the form of a suppository, inserted in the vagina, has shown promise in improving vaginal health and alleviating symptoms. This is a good option for a patient on aromatase inhibitors for the treatment of breast cancer.

- ORAL OSPEMIFENE: Ospemifene, an oral selective estrogen receptor modulator (SERM), is an option for women who prefer oral treatment.

- LUBRICANTS AND MOISTURIZERS: Over-the-counter lubricants and moisturizers can provide relief from dryness. While some contain additives that may be irritating, there are so many options on the market now that you will undoubtedly be able to find one that you tolerate well (see sidebar for more).

- TOPICAL LIDOCAINE: For severe pain during intercourse (known as dyspareunia), topical lidocaine applied to vulvar affected areas before sexual activity can reduce pain.

Vaginal Lubricants and Moisturizers

If you've explored the feminine products aisle at your nearby pharmacy or scrolled through the many options in the online sexual health category, you know there is an overwhelming number of products to choose from (and they all promise the ultimate in sexual pleasure). I can't speak to the legitimacy of all the various product promises, but understanding the difference between the two product categories—lubricants and moisturizers—can help you get what you need.

Vaginal lubricants help reduce friction during sexual activity. *Friction,* in this context, refers to the resistance encountered when one surface or object moves over another. Lubricants make all the difference in situations where friction is high, as they can make sex more comfortable and pleasurable. They can also assist with arousal. To increase comfort, reduce pain, and enhance pleasure, use early on during sex (in this instance, there is such a thing as too little, too late).

Vaginal moisturizers are meant to be used regularly over time and not specifically in the heat of the moment during sexual encounters. Like moisturizers you might apply to your face or legs, these products are designed to add a protective barrier to the vaginal lining. The barrier helps improve moisture and reduce the discomfort associated with vaginal dryness.

When choosing either a vaginal lubricant or moisturizer, be sure to read labels carefully to make sure you're getting the specific type of product you want.

Neither vaginal moisturizers nor lubricants will address the underlying cause of vaginal dryness, especially the cellular changes in vaginal tissue. For addressing such concerns, estrogen therapy and other FDA-approved medications are going to be more effective. Still, even though they don't target the root cause, vaginal moisturizers and lubricants are essential to have in your Menopause Tool Kit if you are dealing with vaginal dryness and want to enhance both comfort and sexual pleasure.

Headaches, see Migraines/Headaches

Heart Palpitations

> It all started with extreme fatigue. My chest would feel so "heavy" at times I thought I was having a heart attack. Then chest palpitations began. My GP sent me to a cardiologist and everything checked out fine with my heart. I was told I was probably dehydrated or was drinking too much coffee. Then, I started having extreme vertigo! I went to an ENT doctor and the tests came back fine, but the vertigo was so bad I had to crawl on the floor. I thought I was having a stroke and at one point my husband had to take me to the ER. A female ER physician did a CT scan of my brain, blood tests for heart attack, etc., but when I told her I was on my period, she suggested the issue might be hormonal. She was the ONLY doctor I had seen in two years that made this connection. A light bulb went off! I could not imagine at forty-five I was having hormonal imbalances or in perimenopause. I did my research and found a doctor who prescribed bioidentical HRT and now I feel amazing.

> —Alayna H.

Forty-two percent of perimenopausal and 52 percent of postmenopausal women report experiencing heart palpitations, which are noticeable alterations in the sensation of your heartbeat. A heart palpitation can be a rapid or irregular heartbeat (arrhythmia); the feeling that your heart has "missed" or "skipped" a beat; or an exaggerated or pounding heartbeat.

Heart palpitations can occur in response to diminishing levels of estrogen, and this hormonal shift has been linked to increases in heart rate, frequency of palpitations, and nonthreatening arrhythmias. Despite this established link, few menopausal patients who visit the doctor with heart palpitations will be told that their changing hormones may be to blame. In fact, palpitations are more likely to be dismissed as a result of stress or anxiety.

To be fair, heart palpitations in menopause should not automatically be blamed on hormones, as there may be underlying issues present. For example, heart palpitations can result from cardiac arrhythmias, and depending on the nature of your palpitations you may need to see a cardiologist to have these ruled out. However, any evaluation that aims to get to the bottom of heart palpitations will ideally include consideration of your age and potential perimenopausal or menopausal status. Menopausal palpitations can cause a great deal of worry, disrupt sleep, bring on depressive symptoms, and disrupt your quality of life. Simply hearing that there is a strong likelihood your hormones are involved could go a long way in lessening the distress associated with heart palpitations.

Strategies for Reducing Heart Palpitations

Far too little research has been done on menopausal heart palpitations, and this has amounted to there being very few fully science-supported approaches to treating or improving them. As with so many areas of menopause, *we need more research* in the area of effective treatments for menopausal heart palpitations.

At the time of this writing, hormone therapy is the only option that has evidence showing it is effective at reducing the prevalence or severity of heart palpitations due to declining estrogen levels. No other treatment options, such as drug therapies, dietary supplements, cognitive-behavioral interventions, or auricular acupressure (also called ear seeding), have been determined to have enough evidence to warrant recommendation.

High Cholesterol/High Triglycerides

I "officially" entered menopause in October 2022 at the age of fifty-six. For the last year I have experienced terrible joint pain despite being at a normal weight, overall healthy, eating a healthful anti-inflammatory diet, and exercising several times a week. My primary care doctor did all sorts of labs including testing for inflammation and rheumatoid arthritis (all results were normal). My cholesterol was high for the first time in my life, and she told me to "continue working" on my already healthful diet. An orthopedic surgeon I saw about my joint pain told me I'm just "unlucky." Neither doctor ever put together that my joint pain or high cholesterol could have anything to do with menopause/lack of estrogen. I have just

started HRT (estradiol patch plus progesterone) and am very hopeful that
my joint pain and cholesterol will improve.

—Beverly W.

Cholesterol is a waxy, fatty substance found in the blood that your body
uses to make hormones, build cell membranes, and metabolize certain vitamins. You need cholesterol to perform these important tasks, but if levels become too high, excess cholesterol can accumulate in your arteries
and potentially lead to blockages. Arterial blockages are a major health
concern, as they can cause heart attack and stroke.

When you get your cholesterol checked by a doctor, they will typically
order a blood test that measures total cholesterol, low-density lipoprotein
(LDL) cholesterol, high-density lipoprotein (HDL) cholesterol, and triglycerides. LDL has been historically referred to as "bad" cholesterol because of its role in creating arterial blockages, and HDL is commonly
known as "good" cholesterol because it helps remove cholesterol from the
blood. In my practice, I will also check apolipoprotein B, which you may
see written as ApoB, and lipoprotein(a), referred to as Lp(a), as these are
more specific for assessing risk of coronary artery disease than the gener-
alized lipid panel. These are tests I would specifically ask for (see chapter 8
for a list of blood tests to discuss with your doctor).

Cholesterol levels often increase sharply in menopause. In my clinic,
most of my menopausal patients are shocked to find an increase in their
lipid panels, with some experiencing as much as a 10–15 percent jump in
LDL and triglyceride levels, despite no significant dietary or exercise
changes. These increases are often attributed to aging alone, but the estrogen decline in menopause has been identified as having an independent
role in altering lipid levels; as estrogen declines, HDL decreases and LDL
and triglycerides increase.

This isn't entirely surprising because there is evidence that shows estrogen is connected to cholesterol levels. In menstruating women, cholesterol
levels rise and fall slightly as estrogen levels change during the monthly

cycle. And because estrogen acts as an antioxidant, when it declines in menopause, LDL particles can more freely oxidize and become more damaging and dangerous to your arteries.

Someday we will know more about how estrogen affects cholesterol, and it seems likely that the details will be found somewhere in the liver. The liver is your body's command center for cholesterol production and metabolism, and liver cells contain estrogen receptors that essentially establish your lipid profile.

The only way to know if you have unhealthy levels of cholesterol is to have your doctor run a lipid panel when you have blood work done. There are no usually noticeable symptoms of abnormal lipids, despite the fact that they may be contributing to narrowing of your arterial walls due to plaque buildup. Ideally, you will want to have your lipid panel run about every five years if they are normal, and more often if they become abnormal.

Strategies for Managing High Cholesterol

NUTRITION

Nutritional strategies include:

- ANTIOXIDANT-RICH DIET: You can help compensate for the loss of estrogen's natural antioxidant impact by eating to maximize antioxidants. Antioxidant-rich foods include green leafy vegetables, such as Swiss chard, spinach, and beet greens; cruciferous vegetables like broccoli and cauliflower; legumes, such as lentils and chickpeas; and squashes, berries, citrus, and dark chocolate.

- DIETARY REGULATION OF OXIDATIVE STRESS: You can also make the dietary choice to avoid foods that increase oxidative stress—which is a large contributor to abnormal lipids. This includes limiting processed meats, deep-fried foods, and sugar-sweetened vegetables.

- FATTY FISH: Getting omega-3 fatty acids from nonfried fatty fish has been linked to a lower risk of coronary heart disease, likely a result of their ability to help lower triglyceride levels. Fatty fish options include sardines, salmon, mackerel, black cod, and bluefin tuna. Higher intake of omega-3 fatty acids over time has also been linked to lower risk of coronary artery disease.

- PROBIOTICS FROM FOOD SOURCES: Research has shown that probiotics can have a significant effect on cholesterol levels and help reduce both triglyceride and LDL levels. Some of the best sources include yogurt, Greek yogurt, buttermilk, cottage cheese, garlic, apple cider vinegar, and fermented or pickled foods, such as sauerkraut and any type of pickled vegetable.

SUPPLEMENTATION

Vitamin D: In postmenopausal women, higher levels of vitamin D have been associated with lower triglycerides, lower body fat, and less incidence of metabolic syndrome. Research has also shown that participants who took vitamin D along with calcium increased vitamin D levels, which correlated with lowered LDL and triglycerides levels, and increased HDL.

It's clear that vitamin D has a lipid-regulating element to it, and we should be sure to keep our levels in the healthy range during menopause. Some guidelines recommend as little as 600–800 IU/day; however, in my practice about 80 percent of my patients are severely deficient in vitamin D. Accordingly, I am currently recommending a daily maintenance dose of 4,000 IU/day (as high as you can go without worries of toxicity) and more by prescription if needed for a clinical deficiency. In my opinion, you should ask to have your vitamin D levels checked every time you have blood work done. See chapter 8 for a full discussion of lab tests to discuss with your doctor. I have created a vitamin D/omega-3/vitamin K combination supplement for my patients—see thepauselife.org for more details.

Omega-3 fatty acids: If you don't regularly consume fatty fish, you can look for an omega-3 fatty acid supplement containing eicosapentaenoic acid (EPA) and docosahexaenoic acid (DHA). Supplemental fish oil has been shown to have a moderate effect on reducing cholesterol levels, and consistent intake has been linked to overall lowered levels of triglycerides.

The lipid-lowering effect of omega-3 fatty acids is consistent if you have normal, high, or borderline high cholesterol.

Berberine: Berberine is a naturally occurring compound found in plants such as goldenseal and barberry. It has long been used in Native American and Chinese medicine to treat a variety of conditions, and research has shown that it can be effective in improving lipid profiles. It's specifically been shown to help lower LDL and triglyceride levels and to increase levels of HDL. It can be purchased as a supplement without a prescription—most of the studies showing benefit were utilizing 500 milligrams once or twice a day. I recommend it to my patients with abnormal lipid profiles.

Fiber: Psyllium is a natural fiber supplement that has shown significant promise in reducing LDL cholesterol and total cholesterol levels. In well-controlled clinical studies involving over 1,500 subjects, psyllium doses ranging from 6 to 15 g/day (most studies used a daily dose of 10 grams) demonstrated substantial reductions in cholesterol levels. The most significant reductions were seen in people with high baseline cholesterol levels. Psyllium can also be a helpful co-therapy when combined with statin drugs and bile acid sequestrants. (If you're looking for a fiber supplement, I have created one for my patients that is available at thepauselife.com that contains psyllium as well as other beneficial grains.)

Pharmacologic Options

Menopausal hormone therapy (MHT) can be helpful in improving your overall lipid profile and in reducing heart disease risk. There are some special considerations when it comes to MHT use for cholesterol-lowering effect:

- If you already have hypertriglyceridemia (high triglycerides), it's important to note that higher doses of oral estrogen may increase triglycerides. For this reason, it may be best for you to use transdermal MHT, a lower oral dose, or a SERM (Selective Estrogen Receptor Modulator) like tibolone.

- The combination of estrogen and a progestogen may be less effective at improving lipid profiles compared to estrogen alone because a progestogen can counteract some of estrogen's beneficial effects on cholesterol levels. However, women with an intact uterus should always take a progestogen with estrogen to protect the endometrial lining.

- According to the timing hypothesis (detailed further in chapter 3 on page 31), MHT use may be safest if it's started before more than ten years have passed since you entered menopause. If it's been ten or more years since you entered menopause, *and* you have significant risk factors for coronary artery disease, you will want to consider having a coronary calcium score test done prior to starting any type of estrogen containing MHT. This test will reveal current arteriosclerosis calcification and can help your doctor determine the safety of MHT use for you.

Lipid-lowering medications: While lifestyle modifications and some supplements can play a pivotal role in managing abnormal lipid profiles during menopause, some women may require lipid-lowering medications. Lipid-lowering medications, especially statins, have been widely prescribed to reduce the risk of cardiovascular disease. However, it's critical to note that statins do not prevent cardiovascular disease or death from cardiovascular disease in women as effectively as they do in men (see sidebar).

Questioning the Value of Statins for Women

Statins have long been considered a powerful tool in helping to lower cholesterol levels and to reduce the risk of cardiovascular disease. These popular medications work by inhibiting an enzyme involved in cholesterol production in the liver, ultimately lowering cholesterol levels in the bloodstream. Statins are a common prescription for high levels of cholesterol, but a recent debate in the medical community has been focused around an important question: Are statins as effective and beneficial for women as they are for men? A definitive conclusion has yet to be reached, but the answer seems to be leaning toward *no*.

- *Survival benefits:* One key point of contention is the impact of statins on overall survival. According to the data in this area, use of statins in women with existing cardiovascular disease or a history of heart attack or stroke (called secondary prevention) has not shown a reduction in overall mortality. The takeaway: Statins don't seem to increase the chances of survival for women in this group.

- *Primary prevention:* Similarly, women without existing cardiovascular disease who take statins (in what's called primary prevention) have not demonstrated an overall mortality benefit or a reduction in cardiovascular events, such as heart attacks and strokes. The takeaway: Statins don't seem to provide significant benefits for healthy women *without* a history of heart disease.

Another consideration in the use of statins is the potentially debilitating side effect of musculoskeletal pain. One of the most common complaints of people taking statins is muscle pain, which may be felt as soreness, tiredness, or weakness in your muscles. The pain can be a mild discomfort, or it can be serious enough to make it hard to do your daily activities. Given that up to 70 percent of women already report experiencing musculoskeletal pain as a side effect of menopause alone, adding a statin to the mix may lead to further discomfort.

I know this leaves the question of statin use open-ended, and if you're already taking one, you may wonder if you should stop. I think for now it's essential to evaluate use on an individual basis. It's clear that statins shouldn't be universally prescribed to all women with high cholesterol, but for some the benefits may outweigh the risks. I hate to sound like a broken record, but we need more research before we can say for sure if statins are the best pharmacologic approach to high cholesterol in women for the prevention of adverse events from cardiovascular disease. You should absolutely discuss this in detail with your own doctor.

Hot Flashes

> I am fifty-two and an emergency physician in a busy, urban level I trauma center. At forty-eight I entered menopause with a few missed periods and then horrible hot flashes that occurred every thirty minutes! I felt this horrible heat and prickly sensation rising from my mid back into my neck and then my scalp until my scalp was soaked with sweat. I actually asked my husband to shave my head once! This also occurred during the early days of the pandemic when I was covered in a cap, masks, and a plastic gown to take care of very sick patients. Most days, I was coated in sweat within minutes of starting my shift. It was awful. But my gynecologist (aka angel) put me on oral HRT and helped adjust it until I felt normal and functional again.
>
> —Stefanie E.

Hot flashes—also called hot *flushes*—are a common menopausal symptom, reported to be experienced by 60–80 percent of women during perimenopause and/or postmenopause. They fall under the category of "vasomotor symptoms." (Another vasomotor symptom, heart palpitations, deserves its own Tool Kit entry. Find it on page 195.) *Vasomotor* means related to constriction or dilation of the blood vessels, although a hot flash actually starts in a region of the brain called the hypothalamus. The hypothalamus is your internal thermostat, and it's very sensitive, requiring a specific balance of different types of neurons to control the body's temperature. This balance is disrupted when estrogen levels decline, leading to a trippy temperature gauge that triggers blood vessels to dilate even when it's not necessary. Blood vessel dilation is what happens to create the hot, flushed sensation of a hot flash to occur. The effect can spread up your chest and onto your face and also make you break into a full sweat. When hot flashes happen at night, they're called night sweats.

Hot flashes are often quoted as the most bothersome symptom of menopause, but based on my experience and research, it's more accurate to describe them as the symptom most *representative* of menopause. That's not to say hot flashes are not bothersome or incredibly annoying and common—they are definitely all of those things—but they've long been the poster symptom of menopause, getting all the attention while less "showy" symptoms that women might experience more get dismissed as merely psychological issues or aging. The issue with hot flashes that *should* be put on a poster is the fact that they can represent increased health risks. Research has linked greater frequency of hot flashes with increased visceral fat gain, and greater severity of hot flashes with elevated risk for cardiovascular disease.

You're likely now wondering how to tell if you are experiencing frequent or severe hot flashes. In the research mentioned, having frequent hot flashes/night sweats was defined as experiencing either of these on six or more days over the course of two weeks. And severity (in a separate study) was defined by asking participants to describe their hot flashes as never, mild, moderate, or severe.

It's not entirely scientifically understood why severe and/or frequent hot flashes are linked to increased health risks. The sleep disturbances that often go hand in hand with night sweats, that is, hot flashes at night, may have something to do with it. Disrupted sleep may indicate reduced levels of melatonin, which have been linked to weight gain in postmenopausal women. Regardless of the reasons for increased risk, if your hot flashes are severe or frequent, it's important to pay attention and be especially proactive in managing them.

Unfortunately, although most women have hot flashes for a few years, some women have them for decades, and reports have shown that the median duration is 7.4 years. They do get better—eventually—with time, but that's a long time to have to endure them.

Here again we are still lacking answers as to why some women have severe hot flashes for many years while others have no hot flashes or mild ones that resolve quickly. If your hot flashes are mild or moderate, you may find relief with some of the lifestyle modifications detailed below. If you have severe hot flashes, you may also benefit from these modifications, but for greater relief you will likely need to consider the addition of a prescription-based medication.

Strategies for Alleviating Hot Flashes

The first strategy for hot flashes is to pay attention. This is important because if you have severe or frequent hot flashes, you may be at increased risk for excess visceral fat gain or heart disease, and you'll want to discuss treatment options and/or other preventative health measures with your doctor ASAP.

To help keep track, consider keeping a hot flash diary like the sample on page 264 in Appendix C. Wherever you keep track, you should "rank" the severity of your hot flashes on the basis of how significantly they disrupt your daily life. You can use this scale:

1 = mild (no interference with usual daily activities)
2 = moderate (interfere with usual daily activities to some extent)
3 = severe (when usual daily activities cannot be performed)

If you notice a lot of 3s, you could be experiencing what might be clinically defined as severe and/or frequent hot flashes, and I suggest making an appointment with your doctor.

Pharmacologic/Therapeutic Options

For treatment of hot flashes, *menopausal hormone therapy* is the gold standard and is considered to be the most effective treatment for vasomotor symptoms. It should be considered the first and best option for menopausal women who are within ten years of their final menstrual periods.

If you are not a candidate for hormone therapy because of a contraindication, other risk factor, or personal preference, there are several non-hormone-based options available. In June 2023, the Menopause Society released a position statement ranking many of these nonhormone options on the basis of the quality and number of scientific studies supporting their use. As a physician who practices evidence-based medicine, I'm thrilled by this because it means you don't have to waste money and time sorting through all the products or practices that falsely promise "fast relief from your hot flashes!"—you can start first with those that have some science supporting their effectiveness.

According to the Menopause Society, there is good and consistent scientific evidence to support the following nonhormone-based treatments for hot flashes:

- COGNITIVE-BEHAVIORAL THERAPY: The body of literature supports the use of CBT in the reduction of hot flashes.

- CLINICAL HYPNOSIS: Hypnosis has been studied for the treatment of hot flashes in two trials. In both trials, clinical hypnosis was significantly better at reducing hot flashes than no treatment.

- SELECTIVE SEROTONIN REUPTAKE INHIBITORS/SEROTONIN-NOREPINEPHRINE REUPTAKE INHIBITORS: SSRIs and SNRIs are associated with mild to moderate improvements in vasomotor symptoms. Only paroxetine is FDA approved at 7.5 mg/day for the treatment of hot flashes.

- GABAPENTIN (NEURONTIN): Gabapentin is associated with improvements in the frequency and severity of vasomotor symptoms.

- FEZOLINETAN: Issued under the brand name Veozah, this medication was granted FDA approval in 2023 for the treatment of hot flashes. It works by inhibiting the neuronal activity that sends out heat signals and triggers hot flashes. While a promising medication, it's currently very expensive and not typically covered by insurance.

There is less research proving the effectiveness of oxybutynin, an antispasmodic medication designed to treat overactive bladder. However, the science that has been done found that women taking oxybutynin experienced a 70–86 percent reduction in hot flashes. The participant group in this study included breast cancer survivors who were receiving tamoxifen or aromatase inhibitors.

NUTRITION

While TMS did not recommend lifestyle interventions for the treatment of hot flashes, such as incorporating specific foods or engaging in certain types of exercise, some studies show some lifestyle modifications may be helpful. For example, a 2022 study published in the journal *Menopause* revealed findings that a reduced-fat vegan diet that included daily soybean intake significantly reduced frequency and severity of hot flashes, helped relieve other physical and sexual symptoms associated with menopause, and produced significant weight loss. Because researchers combined the vegan component with daily soybean consumption, it's impossible to say which part of the dietary intervention was most effective—but what I like about this study is that it demonstrates the potential for dietary strategies to produce noticeable improvements.

If you can be consistent with lifestyle habits that promote good health, this may influence the severity of your hot flashes. Keeping your blood sugar, blood pressure, and cholesterol levels in check and not smoking can go a long way toward establishing the kind of metabolic health that could benefit your experience of menopause. Unfortunately, there's no guarantee that you'll be rewarded for your efforts specifically with less severe hot flashes (or other menopausal symptoms), but investments in good health will always be worth it.

Incontinence, see Genitourinary Syndrome

Insulin Resistance

> Perimenopause began for me while I was in pharmacy school. The brain fog made me think I was losing my mind (perhaps even early dementia). My inability to recall information led a preceptor to tell me they didn't think that I could pass my boards. I found menopause-tok & began doing my own research. I approached an ob-gyn who dismissed me and my concerns due to the results of blood tests. She told me that my long list of peri-menopause symptoms was all due to a slight increase in A1c. Never mind that insulin insensitivity is common in menopause. I did more research and then approached my PCP (who is aware of my high health literacy). This appointment went better primarily because I had found a combina-tion of supplements that had already begun to return my brain function

and helped me to begin feeling like my old self. Since then I have passed my boards (after a couple failed attempts) but I am now feeling that my supplements aren't the entire answer but I'm not sure where to turn now.

—Jessica T.

Insulin resistance (IR) is what happens when your cells become less sensitive to insulin, a hormone secreted by the pancreas that is essential to glucose (blood sugar) metabolism. When your cells don't respond to insulin, it can result in consistently high levels of blood sugar, a risk factor for both type 2 diabetes and chronic low-grade inflammation.

As I mentioned in chapter 6, declining estrogen levels in and around menopause put us at a greater risk of developing insulin resistance. Estrogen assists in glucose metabolism a couple of ways—by helping your muscle tissue use glucose as fuel and by suppressing gluconeogenesis, the production of glucose in the liver. As we lose estrogen we lose its involvement in metabolic processes, and this can leave us vulnerable to dysfunction in our cells' ability to use and store fuel from food and to perpetually high blood sugar.

There aren't any obvious symptoms of insulin resistance to watch out for, but there are established risk factors, including:

- age forty-five and over

- a family history of type 2 diabetes

- obesity, and especially abdominal obesity (visceral fat)

- being physically inactive

- high blood pressure and/or high cholesterol

- polycystic ovarian syndrome (PCOS)

- sleep apnea

- fatty liver disease

- use of certain blood pressure medications, steroids, and those used to treat psychiatric disorders or HIV

- Cushing's disease and hypothyroidism

It's important to pay attention to your personal risk factors for insulin resistance because if left untreated, IR can lead to prediabetes and then type 2 diabetes. Type 2 diabetes is associated with increased risk for serious health issues, including stroke, heart disease, kidney and eye disease, and diabetic neuropathy.

Strategies for Correcting Insulin Resistance

To treat and reduce your risk for insulin resistance, you must prioritize healthy lifestyle choices that maximize your body's metabolic potential. These choices will focus on eating and exercising strategically to support your cells' sensitivity to insulin. You want cells that are sensitive to insulin—the opposite of resistant—because this translates to balanced blood sugar and low levels of inflammation. You can go a long way toward protecting yourself from some of the most common chronic diseases by incorporating habits that promote insulin sensitivity. I'll share with you some of the best habits below.

NUTRITION

There are two key nutritional goals you can aim for that will help protect your metabolic health during menopause and beyond. (These nutritional goals form the foundation of *The Galveston Diet*, my program and book designed for menopausal women.)

Eat foods with a low glycemic index score: The glycemic index is a tool that measures how quickly a food makes your blood sugar rise. Foods lower on the glycemic index produce a slower rise in blood sugar, which is better for your metabolism, mood (no blood sugar "crashes"), and more. Foods low on the glycemic index include vegetables, fruits, whole-grain products, nuts, lean meats, and beans.

Get a minimum of 25 grams of fiber per day: Daily dietary fiber intake has been shown in research to help reduce fasting blood sugar and insulin levels. Both soluble fiber products and fiber from natural foods are effective at improving blood sugar management and insulin sensitivity.

Some of the best fiber sources (as also elaborated upon in *The Galveston Diet*) include beans, broccoli, berries, avocado (my fave), chia seeds, pumpkin seeds, artichoke, edamame, squash, greens, whole oats, corn, spelt, quinoa, sunflower seeds, banana, apples, bran, almonds, sweet potatoes, prunes, and more.

When you eat foods low on the glycemic index and get enough fiber each day, you will by default help your body stay on track to achieve and maintain a healthy body composition.

Incorporate plenty of polyphenols into your diet. Polyphenols are beneficial compounds found in plants that have awesome antioxidant activity. Some of the best sources include:

apples

berries

broccoli

carrots

chili peppers

cumin

dark chocolate (because cocoa is a major source of polyphenols)

flax seeds

SUPPLEMENTATION

Some supplements can help support dietary efforts to improve insulin sensitivity. These include:

- MAGNESIUM: Many studies looking at different types of magnesium supplementation have shown benefit: Magnesium in various forms, 250–360 mg of elemental Mg++ per day, all showed benefit.

- ZINC: Zinc deficiency is clearly associated with increasing risk of insulin resistance, but supplementation for a woman who does not have a zinc deficiency has mixed results.

- VITAMIN C: Research has suggested that vitamin C levels are associated with metabolic syndrome, but we need more studies to find the exact dosage for benefit.

- PROBIOTICS: Use of probiotics was linked to improved insulin resistance scores in menopausal women; supplements should contain *Lactobacillus* and *Bifidobacterium* species.

While not as effective as the others mentioned above, vitamin D was also found to introduce noticeable positive changes in glucose metabolism.

PHYSICAL ACTIVITY

Regular physical exercise is incredibly important to improving insulin sensitivity. In fact, just thirty minutes of exercise at least five days a week can improve your cells' responsiveness to insulin and increase "glucose uptake," which simply means that your tissues use more glucose, leaving less to sit in the bloodstream where it can begin to cause problems.

PHARMACOLOGIC OPTIONS

As we discussed in chapter 6, MHT seems to be effective.

Irregular Heartbeat, see Heart Palpitations

Irritability, see Mental Health Disorders and Mood Changes

Irritable Bowel Syndrome, see Gastrointestinal Issues

Itchy Ears, see Skin Changes

Itchy Skin, see Skin Changes

Joint Pain, see Muskuloskeletal Pain

Kidney Stones

Kidney stones are painful mineral deposits in the kidneys. In 2023, groundbreaking research came out suggesting a correlation between estrogen levels and kidney stone disease, shedding light on a potential breakthrough in managing the condition. Interestingly, the research found that higher levels of estrogen may be linked to a reduced risk of kidney stone disease. To understand why, we need to look at how estrogen affects a critical player in this scenario: a protein called PAT1.

PAT1 is a protein found in the kidney that helps move negatively charged ions across cell membranes. One of these negatively charged ions, oxalate, is a significant component of kidney stones. When estrogen is in the picture, it appears to slow activity of PAT1, leading to a decrease in the transport of oxalate. What this means is that estrogen seems to reduce the formation of kidney stones by making it more challenging for minerals to accumulate in the kidneys.

The connection between estrogen and kidney stones isn't just about preventing painful stones; it also relates to optimal kidney function. Estrogen's ability to fine-tune PAT1 appears to help balance negatively charged ions in the body, and maintaining this balance is crucial for ensuring that the kidneys work correctly and effectively.

Strategies for Addressing Kidney Stones

The research in this area is so new that we don't have any evidence-based strategies yet. The exciting thing is that attention is being paid to the significance of estrogen deprivation in women's health—we will only continue to know more in the future! For now, be sure to discuss your hormonal status with your physician if you are dealing with kidney stones.

Memory Issues, see Brain Fog

Menstrual Cycle Changes

I had always had what I would call a clockwork cycle, same time, same day every cycle, until suddenly they started becoming heavier and more frequent. The heavy bleeding turned into bleeding approximately 70 percent of the year. I decided this wasn't normal and went to see my doctor, who agreed it was not. He immediately booked me in for an ultrasound. The result came back as "unexplainable bleeding." I had a proactive ob-gyn, who ran through my options, and we agreed that my first step should be an IUD (Mirena). Within two months I was period free. Two years later, I have several months of sleepless nights due to hot flashes, or as I like to say "going thermal." My doctor did blood work and informed me that I was technically postmenopausal and gave me options to assist with my symptoms. I am now on HRT estradiol patches, and symptoms are improving slowly. I am thankful I have a doctor that does not dismiss me and that I educated myself regarding menopause. I know we should not have to suffer in silence.

—Tracy E.

As a result of the hormonal fluctuations that occur during perimenopause, most women will experience some degree of menstrual irregularity during the menopausal transition. But *most* does not mean *all*—15–25 percent of women report minimal or no change in menstrual regularity prior to their final menstrual period.

If you are lucky enough to have or have had reliable periods, some of the noticeable changes in your monthly cycle may help predict how close you are to menopause. Generally, once you have gone sixty days or more without a period, you are likely to enter menopause within two years. I do want to emphasize the word *generally* here because menopause doesn't always follow the rules and can't always be easily categorized.

Here is a list of the variety of menstrual changes you may experience as your hormones begin to change:

- HEAVIER PERIODS: These are caused by fluctuations in estrogen and progesterone and are more likely in the late transition. They are more common in obese women and in women with fibroids.

- LIGHTER PERIODS: These are caused by decreasing hormone levels.

- LONGER CYCLES: Shifting hormones can disrupt the regularity of ovulation and lead to more time between periods. Longer cycles are more likely to occur in late perimenopause.

- SHORTER CYCLES: Shifting hormones can also lead to less time between periods. Shorter cycles are more common in early perimenopause.

- IRREGULAR SPOTTING: Light bleeding that occurs between periods, aka spotting, is common in perimenopause and happens as a result of hormone fluctuations.

- MISSED PERIODS: These happen when your ovaries stop releasing eggs regularly, or in pregnancy.

- CHANGES IN MENSTRUAL SYMPTOMS: Intensity of cramps and PMS symptoms may change.

It's very common for any of the changes noted on this list to be caused by hormonal fluctuations. But that doesn't mean hormonal fluctuations are the cause of abnormal uterine bleeding 100 percent of the time. For this reason, if and when menstrual irregularities begin to occur, it's really important that you see a gynecologist. Ideally, this doctor will be someone who really listens to you and can help you distinguish harmful symptoms from those that might be just annoying. (To help your doctor best identify what could be going on, I recommend keeping a symptom journal before your appointment. See Appendix C for a template.)

If your reproductive years have been relatively free from gynecological drama, you might be inclined to think you can manage any menstrual changes without medical support. However, it's vitally important that you not try to ride out any kind of excessive, unusually heavy, or prolonged bleeding, especially if it's accompanied by pain or other symptoms. This can be indicative of underlying issues, such as adenomyosis, fibroids, polyps, or hyperplasia. Please know that if tests indicate these conditions, there is no automatic or established medical need for an immediate hysterectomy or oophorectomy. Other options such as progestin IUD insertion or endometrial ablation may be available to you. If your doctor suggests that the only option is removal of your uterus or ovaries or both, I strongly encourage you to get a second opinion; surgical menopause has drastic consequences, and you don't want to enter into it unless it's absolutely necessary.

If it's been one year or more since your last period and you are postmenopausal, any vaginal bleeding is considered abnormal and should be evaluated. If you started hormone therapy less than six months ago, your bleeding may be a result of your body adjusting to MHT, but you should still report your symptoms to your doctor.

Strategies for Perimenopausal Menstrual Changes

You will want to see your gynecologist for the strategy or treatment that's best for you. Here are some of the options that may be recommended:

- EXPECTANT MANAGEMENT is defined as watchful waiting or close monitoring by medical professionals instead of immediate treatment.

- HORMONAL MEDICATIONS, such as oral contraceptives, progestogens, or hormone-releasing intrauterine devices (IUDs), can help regulate the menstrual cycle and reduce abnormal bleeding.

- NONSTEROIDAL ANTI-INFLAMMATORY DRUGS (NSAIDS, LIKE ASPIRIN OR IBUPROFEN) can help relieve pain and actually reduce bleeding during menstruation.

- ANTIFIBRINOLYTICS, such as tranexamic acid, help counteract heavy menstrual bleeding that can be caused by an increase in fibrinolysis, your body's natural anticlotting process.

- DILATATION AND CURETTAGE (D&C) may be performed to remove abnormal uterine tissue if it's determined to be the cause of your heavy bleeding.

- ENDOMETRIAL ABLATION uses heat, cold, laser, or electricity to permanently destroy the uterine lining, reducing or stopping menstrual bleeding.

- HYSTERECTOMY may be recommended in the most severe cases or when other treatments have failed, but rarely, if ever, as a first course of action. Though a hysterectomy means the removal of the uterus, the procedure also cuts off blood supply to your ovaries, which in turn hastens their decline in function. This is why hysterectomy can put a woman into menopause on average about 4.4 years sooner than if the uterus were intact.

If you are *postmenopausal* and you are experiencing bleeding, it's very important that you be evaluated to rule out endometrial or cervical cancer or atrophic vaginitis/GSM. Atrophic vaginitis is a common cause of postmenopausal bleeding and, if diagnosed, will be treated with topical estrogen therapy or lubricants/moisturizers.

Mental Health Disorders and Mood Changes

At forty-five, I began having inexplicable anxiety. This was accompanied by flooding periods, insomnia, dizziness, palpitations, digestive problems, and restless leg syndrome. My gynecologist said I was anemic from heavy bleeding. This explained some of what was happening, but I know now I was also in perimenopause. When I asked about the other symptoms I was having, she literally pointed to her midsection and said, "I only deal with this, not *this*," and gestured to her heart and head. This led me on a long, isolated, and dark journey to figure out what was "wrong" with me. Instead of answers, doctors gave me antidepressants, Xanax, and a prescription for a therapist. I was defeated. There were times I wanted to die. I had to find my own answers and be my own advocate. It took five years, thousands of hours of research, and finally MHT to finally come back to myself again. I am forever scarred by that time of my life and by the way I was treated by doctors and the way they dismissed me.

—Amy P.

While menopause is caused by the physical change of ovarian failure, it can also bring about a lot of psychological change. Research has consistently shown that entering menopause comes with an elevated risk of experiencing mental health issues such as depression and anxiety, and that shifts in mood, cognition, and emotional well-being are common. The symptoms can range from mild to severe and can significantly affect your overall quality of life.

In a lot of ways, we don't really understand why women are more susceptible to mental health challenges during specific stages of life, including menopause (yes, we need more research!). But some scientific insight has suggested that it may involve the concept of "biological vulnerability windows." These are periods of heightened vulnerability to mood disorders that may be "opened" during significant hormonal fluctuations, such as the menstrual cycle, pregnancy, postpartum, and, notably, the menopausal transition. Certainly there are other factors involved because not all women who pass through these periods of vulnerability will develop mood disorders or experience profound changes in emotional well-being. But for some women, hormonal fluctuations can remarkably disrupt mental health and wellness.

The heightened vulnerability to mood changes and mood disorders in menopause most likely has a great deal to do with the decline of estrogen. Estrogen helps regulate the activity of the neurotransmitters serotonin, dopamine, and norepinephrine, which are linked to depression and mood. There are also estrogen receptors throughout the brain. In both cases, as estrogen declines, metabolic and neurological functions that are dependent upon estrogen are undoubtedly altered.

Strategies for Dealing with Mental Health Disorders and Mood Changes

To be absolutely clear: I am not a mental health professional, and the strategies listed here are not intended to replace psychological treatment offered by a therapist, psychologist, or psychiatrist.

If you are ever having thoughts of hurting yourself or others, this is an emergency and you should seek help immediately from an emergency department. You can also get help by calling SAMHSA's National Helpline at 1-800-662-HELP (4357). This is a free, confidential, 24/7, 365-day-a-year treatment referral and information service (in English and Spanish) for individuals and families facing mental and/or substance use disorders.

Mental health challenges that arise during menopause should never be approached with an "I'll just grit my teeth and get through it" attitude, not when there are available and effective treatments and protocols that can produce life-changing improvements in mood and mood disorders. If you are experiencing noticeable and prolonged changes in your mental health,

I encourage you to seek out a mental health professional for help. You can also explore the various interventions mentioned here, including hormone therapy, omega-3 fatty acids, and botanical supplements.

PHARMACOLOGIC OPTIONS

Estrogen therapy has not been FDA approved for the treatment of mood disorders, but it *has* been shown to have psychological benefits and may help:

- REDUCE SYMPTOMS OF DEPRESSION. Hormonal therapy, particularly estrogen-based interventions, has been found to have effects similar to classic antidepressant agents, such as SSRIs and SNRIs. Estrogens, specifically estradiol, have shown antidepressant properties.

- PREVENT DEPRESSION IN PERIMENOPAUSE. In perimenopause, estradiol is found to be preventative for the new onset of depressive disorders—meaning, a woman treated with estrogen during perimenopause is less likely to develop new-onset depressive disorders. One randomized trial involving 172 women explored the effectiveness of estrogen administration, specifically transdermal estradiol (0.1 mg/day) combined with intermittent oral micronized progesterone (200 mg/day for twelve days every three months), versus a placebo. After one year, women who received estrogens plus progesterone were significantly less likely to exhibit depressive symptoms compared to those who received a placebo. The effect was more pronounced in women in the early perimenopausal stage.

- SERVE AS ADJUNCTIVE THERAPY FOR DEPRESSION IN POSTMENOPAUSE (IN ADDITION TO AN ANTIDEPRESSANT). Estrogen therapy is currently considered ineffective as a treatment alone for depressive disorders in postmenopausal women and should not be considered a replacement or alternative to an antidepressant in postmenopause; however, it may help lessen symptoms and can boost the clinical effectiveness of an antidepressant.

- PREVENT THE ONSET OF DEPRESSIVE SYMPTOMS IN WOMEN: Estrogen therapy, in the form of transdermal estradiol, when combined with intermittent micronized progesterone may prevent the onset of depressive symptoms in nondepressed perimenopausal women.

- ENHANCE MOOD AND IMPROVE WELL-BEING. Evidence has found that estrogen therapy enhances mood and improves well-being in nondepressed perimenopausal women.

SUPPLEMENTATION

Certain supplements, including botanical ones, have been evaluated for their potential to alleviate mood and anxiety changes during menopause. Some of the most promising options are:

- ST. JOHN'S WORT: St. John's wort, a plant traditionally used for its antidepressant properties, has shown effectiveness in treating mild to moderate depression. It is believed to work by increasing the levels of neurotransmitters like serotonin and dopamine in the brain.

- BLACK COHOSH: Black cohosh, a plant used for various women's health issues, has been found to reduce symptoms of menopause. By binding to estrogen receptors and reducing luteinizing hormone levels, it can alleviate menopausal-related mood changes.

- GINSENG: While we need more research on ginseng, a root used in traditional Chinese medicine, it may be beneficial for mood and anxiety changes during menopause, as it has shown promise in improving overall well-being and helping the body cope with stress.

- KAVA: Kava, a South Pacific plant, has potential in reducing anxiety in peri- and postmenopausal women. It works by increasing GABA levels in the brain, promoting relaxation. The active ingredient in kava is kavalactones, and effective dosage begins at 70 mg/day but should not exceed 250 mg/day due to potential toxicity.

- OMEGA-3 FATTY ACIDS (N-3 PUFA): Omega-3 fatty acids have been studied for their role in improving emotional and cognitive behaviors during menopause transition. Eicosapentaenoic acid (EPA) is one of several omega-3 fatty acids. It is found in cold-water fatty fish, such as salmon. It is also found in fish oil supplements, along with docosahexaenoic acid (DHA). Studies have shown that up to 2 grams of EPA daily can reduce symptoms of major depression, bipolar disorder, schizophrenia, anxiety disorders, and ADHD.

Migraines/Headaches

A migraine is a type of headache often characterized by intense throbbing pain on one side of the head. Migraines affect women disproportionately and occur most often during midlife. There are two main types of migraines:

1. *Migraine without aura:* This is the most common type and lacks the neurological symptoms or "aura" that precede a migraine attack.

2. *Migraine with aura:* This type is characterized by neurological symptoms that occur before or at the onset of a migraine, such as visual disturbances, speech problems, numbness, tingling, or weakness. (If you experience migraines with aura and have questions about the use of MHT, I recommend you read the sidebar on page 222.)

These potentially debilitating and painful headaches are often associated with hormonal fluctuations. They tend to start around the time of menarche (your first period), and many women will experience menstrual migraines, which are migraines that are closely associated with their menstrual cycles. These migraines may occur just before, during, or after menstruation. Other women will experience an increase in or a worsening of migraines during the menopausal transition. And still others may experience only menstrual migraines and find complete resolution of them during menopause. In all of these cases, it seems clear that estrogen fluctuations play some role in triggering or alleviating migraines. Researchers have theorized that women with migraines may experience a faster decline in estrogen levels during the menopause transition, making them more susceptible to hormonal migraines.

Strategies for Dealing with Migraines

The relationship between migraines and menopause is complex, with hormonal fluctuations playing a significant role in triggering or alleviating these headaches. I recommend consulting your doctor for a personalized treatment plan, which may include some of the strategies mentioned here. Ultimately, you may find that a combination approach works best for symptom relief.

Supplementation options include some nonprescription *neutraceuticals*, such as magnesium, riboflavin (vitamin B2), butterbur, feverfew, and coenzyme Q10, which have demonstrated potential in preventing migraines and may reduce the frequency and severity of migraine attacks.

Pharmacologic options include:

- ABORTIVE THERAPY: These treatments focus on relieving acute migraine pain when it occurs. Common abortive treatments include prescriptions such as triptans, nonsteroidal anti-inflammatory drugs (NSAIDs), and antiemetics to combat nausea and vomiting.

- PREVENTIVE THERAPY: For individuals with frequent or severe migraines, preventive therapy may be recommended. Medications such as beta-blockers, tricyclic antidepressants (TCAs), anticonvulsants, and certain blood pressure medications have shown effectiveness.

- MENOPAUSAL HORMONE THERAPY: MHT is not FDA approved for migraine treatment or prevention, but some doctors consider its use in premenopausal and perimenopausal women to stabilize falling estrogen levels, which may relieve migraines that are triggered by estrogen decline.

- THERAPIES ON THE HORIZON: Emerging treatments targeting calcitonin gene-related peptide (CGRP), a neuropeptide associated with migraines, are being developed. These monoclonal antibody therapies may prove to be very effective for migraine treatment.

Migraines with Aura and Menopausal Hormone Therapy

If you get visual disturbances, speech problems, or numbness or tingling in the extremities before or during a migraine, that's called migraine with aura. Women with a history of migraines, especially those with aura, have been cautioned against using MHT because of concerns about stroke risk. But is this really the case for all women with migraines? Let's review.

Historically, the use of estrogens (usually in the form of contraceptive agents) was associated with a slight but present dose-dependent increased risk of arteriolar blood clots, such as found in stroke. Because of this concern, women with migraines and particularly those with aura were often discouraged from using MHT. Recent research, however, has shed light on this issue and challenged the notion that all women with migraines are at equal risk when using MHT.

It is important to note that any form of systemic estrogen can *slightly* increase the risk of arteriolar clotting as found in strokes due to "sticky platelets," but especially in patients taking high doses of estrogen as found in high-dose birth control pills and especially those with pre-existing risk factors such as atherosclerotic disease and a history of smoking. Since the increased risk of stroke appears to be dose dependent and traditional MHT is much lower dosing than the estrogen levels found in contraception, it makes sense that the stroke risk for MHT dosing would be increasingly diminished.

It's crucial to recognize that not all women with migraines, even those with aura, have the same risk profile for arteriolar blood clots. Assessing individual risk factors, such as age, smoking status, and other medical conditions, is essential when considering MHT.

Ultimately, if you have a history of migraines, with or without aura, and you have no other risk factors for clotting issues, you should not be automatically excluded from MHT. But you will want to find a doctor with whom you can work closely to discuss and develop a plan for hormone therapy. This doctor will ideally help you select the most appropriate form of estrogen therapy (if for you the benefits outweigh the risks) and closely monitor you for potential side effects.

Mood Changes, see Mental Health Disorders and Mood Changes

Muscle Aches, see Musculoskeletal Pain

Muscle Loss, see Sarcopenia

Musculoskeletal Pain

I am a fifty-two-year-old mother of two and I work as an occupational therapist with children with special needs. I never had a problem doing the physical requirements of my job such as picking up small children from their chairs to work with them on the floor or running with children in the hallways. In my late forties, my period started to become irregular, and I was gaining weight and physically slowing down. My ob-gyn did a few tests to rule out other diagnoses and I was officially diagnosed with perimenopause. The hardest part was that my body just hurt. In my joints and especially in my muscles to the point where I had severe muscle spasms and pelvic pain. This pain was frequently occurring right before my menstrual cycle. I couldn't exercise and coworkers had to help me with the physical demands of my job. Then the hot flashes and sleepless nights started. Even my eczema that I hadn't had since I was a teenager flared up. I felt like I was falling apart.

—Karen C.

Musculoskeletal pain (MSP) is a singular term for a collection of symptoms that can include muscle pain, joint pain (arthralgia), joint inflammation (arthritis), and frozen shoulder. Frozen shoulder has its own distinct list of treatment options, so I've created a separate entry for it that you'll find on page 184.

MSP is one of the most bothersome symptoms I see in my patients, and it is a frequently reported complaint on social media. The pain of MSP is rampant, and so too is the frustration, as symptoms are often dismissed as "just a part of getting older" or misdiagnosed as fibromyalgia (see page 225 for a sidebar of fibromyalgia and menopause).

MSP can develop at any point in menopause, but it's especially prevalent in perimenopause; some reports show that just over *70 percent* of perimenopausal women deal with MSP. In postmenopause, women are also at higher risk of experiencing an uptick in the pain level to what we doctors describe as moderate to severe musculoskeletal pain. It's not entirely understood why there is such a profound increase in MSP during the menopausal transition and in postmenopause, but given the timing of the reported increase in symptoms, we can logically assume that hormonal shifts are primarily to blame. Plus, we've seen that MHT is effective at reducing the frequency and severity of joint pain associated with menopausal transitions.

Here's a little more on how the symptoms of MSP may be presented:

- ARTHRALGIA: Arthralgia refers to pain in one or more joints without clinical signs of inflammation or underlying joint disease. Studies have shown that arthralgia is present in at least 50 percent of women around the time of menopause, with around 21 percent of women reporting this as the *most troublesome symptom of menopause.* These arthralgias may also be accompanied by muscle pain, fatigue, mood changes, sleep disturbances, weight gain, anxiety, and/or stress.

- ARTHRITIS: Unlike arthralgia, arthritis involves clinical signs of joint inflammation or an underlying pathological abnormality. It's important to differentiate between arthralgia and arthritis because the treatments can be different. You will want to report the specifics of your joint pain symptoms to your doctor so that they can assess and exclude the possibility of early arthritis or another underlying inflammatory rheumatic disorder.

Fibromyalgia and Menopause

Fibromyalgia is a chronic condition that causes pain all over the body, including musculoskeletal pain, and other symptoms such as fatigue, depression and anxiety, and memory issues. These same symptoms may also occur in response to menopausal hormone changes; the difference is that the origin of fibromyalgia is believed to be related to an issue with the central nervous system's processing of pain rather than hormonal fluctuations. However, because the symptoms can be very similar, researchers have theorized that menopausal musculoskeletal pain is often misdiagnosed as fibromyalgia, and that estrogen deficiency may also play a role in the development of fibromyalgia. The data strongly supports this theory.

When researchers looked at one hundred patients with primary fibromyalgia, two key factors overlapped with the diagnosis of menopausal hormone changes: (1) Women were the predominant gender affected, and (2) the average age at which fibromyalgia symptoms began was around forty-six years old (right around perimenopause). Interestingly, of the one hundred patients, sixty-five of them had gone into menopause before being diagnosed with fibromyalgia, and the average age of menopause was forty-two years (much earlier than the typical average of fifty-one). Also notable: Many of the women experienced surgically induced menopause and did not receive sufficient estrogen therapy. From these statistics, it seemed clear that—at least in this participant group—changes in estrogen were in some way associated with the onset of fibromyalgia.

Other research has identified estrogen deficiency as a significant contributing factor in the development of fibromyalgia and has shown that estrogen therapy may help relieve symptoms for select patients.

Strategies for Reducing Musculoskeletal Pain

First off, if you are experiencing symptoms of musculoskeletal pain, whatever you do, do something—you don't have to sit back and suffer through what can be debilitating and disruptive pain. Second, whatever strategy you select, be sure to be consistent with it, as the lessening of symptom severity may not be immediately noticeable.

Here are some strategies for minimizing symptoms of MSP.

NUTRITION

Consuming an anti-inflammatory diet rich in fruits, vegetables, lean proteins, and healthy fats can help reduce inflammation and joint pain. Avoiding processed and refined foods, artificial additives, and excessive alcohol can also keep inflammation down.

EXERCISE

Regular physical activity helps keep joints lubricated and maintains joint health. If you are experiencing joint pain, consider trying low-impact exercises such as yoga or swimming. Also, be sure to incorporate stretch breaks or short walks or bursts of activity throughout your day to help lessen stiffness and increase circulation.

SUPPLEMENTATION

Omega-3 fatty acids and fiber supplements can help reduce inflammation and improve overall joint health. Additionally, natural compounds like turmeric and resveratrol have shown promise in managing joint pain.

PHARMACOLOGIC OPTIONS

Menopausal hormone therapy (MHT) has been linked to reductions in joint pain and stiffness and may be beneficial for women experiencing severe joint pain during menopause. It should be noted that in one study the prevalence of joint pain or stiffness and general aches and pains was double in women who discontinued MHT compared to those who discontinued placebo.

NSAIDs (nonsteroidal anti-inflammatory drugs), such as ibuprofen, naproxen, and aspirin, are successful in limiting the pain and inflammation in MSP but should be used for short-term issues only.

Night Sweats, see Hot Flashes

Nonalcoholic Fatty Liver Disease (NAFLD)

Nonalcoholic fatty liver disease (NAFLD) is a condition in which excessive fat builds up in your liver cells. If left untreated, it can progress to the more advanced nonalcoholic steatohepatitis (NASH), cirrhosis, or liver cancer. As its name suggests, NAFLD is not related to alcohol consumption; liver damage or disease caused by heavy alcohol use is referred to as alcoholic liver disease.

NAFLD has become more prevalent in women in recent years, and research has shown that if you are postmenopausal, you are 2.4 times more likely to develop nonalcoholic fatty liver disease than if you are premenopausal. This increase in risk is believed to be due in part to the loss of estrogen, which predisposes menopausal women to gain visceral fat. As you may remember from chapter 6, this is the kind of belly fat that sits deep in the abdominal cavity, close to your liver and other vital organs. Visceral fat is a metabolic disruptor that tends to interfere in organ function and can contribute to fat accumulation in the liver. If more than 5–10 percent of the liver becomes fat, nonalcoholic fatty liver disease is likely to develop.

Additional factors that may put you at increased risk of developing NAFLD include:

- high levels of free testosterone, bioavailable testosterone, and free androgen index (naturally high or through the use of a testosterone replacement; see note on Biote pellets on page 102)

- vitamin D deficiency

- surgical menopause

- type 2 diabetes

- obesity

- insulin resistance

- metabolic syndrome

- high intake of fructose-sweetened beverages, such as sodas

Strategies for Reducing Risk of NAFLD

NUTRITION

You can reduce your risk of nonalcoholic fatty liver disease by taking steps to maintain normal lipid, glucose, and insulin levels. Eating a diet that is low in added sugars and rich in fiber and antioxidants, especially foods rich in vitamin D (fatty fish, mushrooms) and vitamin E (nuts, seeds, and some vegetable oils), can help keep these levels in the healthy range. More research is needed to determine the optimal dosage and duration of vitamin D supplementation for NAFLD patients, so it's best to try to get it from food sources.

SUPPLEMENTATION

In people who have developed NAFLD, the following supplements (when combined with a healthy diet and exercise) may help improve liver health because of their antioxidant and anti-inflammatory properties and by reducing inflammation and protecting against additional liver damage:

- VITAMIN E (THE MOST STUDIED): in the form of tocopherol, 800 IU/day has been demonstrated in multiple studies to improve the structure and function of the liver as well as decrease the risk of death from NAFLD

- SILIMARIN/MILK THISTLE: 420–450 mg/day containing the Eurosil 85 formulation

- OMEGA-3 FATTY ACIDS: 4 g/day was the average dose in the studies

- COENZYME Q10: 100 mg/day

- BERBERINE: 0.3–1.5 g/day; all doses showed a benefit

- CURCUMIN/TURMERIC: 500 mg/day combined with piperine for increased absorption (I have created a turmeric supplement for my patients and students, see thepauselife.com for details.)

PHYSICAL ACTIVITY

Engaging in regular physical activity is essential to your overall metabolic health, which benefits liver and other organ function.

When researchers looked at what kind of exercise was most effective in reducing risk of NAFLD, they found that individuals who engaged in 150 or more minutes per week of physical activity and those who completed two or more strength-based workouts per week had a lower risk of NAFLD.

PHARMACOLOGIC OPTIONS

Even with healthy habits in place, decreasing estrogen levels may put you at risk of visceral fat gain and increased fat accumulation in the liver, which can lead to NAFLD. Research has shown that hormone therapy may have a protective effect against NAFLD in postmenopausal women, even if metabolic syndrome is present. Transdermal therapy (delivered via a patch) *specifically* may be the most beneficial for preventing the development and halting the progression of NAFLD.

Osteoporosis

Osteoporosis is a progressive bone disease that leads to thin, brittle, and weak bones, putting you at increased risk for fracture. In chapter 6, I discussed the gender bias of osteoporosis, which is obvious from this stat alone: Women are four times as likely to develop osteoporosis as men. The primary reason for this discrepancy is the loss of estrogen in menopause, which is considered the most common cause of osteoporosis. Osteoporosis happens because the process of bone remodeling, which is like a continuous renovation of your bones, gets out of balance. Normally, your body removes old, weak bone tissue and replaces it with fresh, strong bone. But in menopause, because of estrogen deprivation and potentially a decline in testosterone levels, this remodeling process is disrupted, and more old bone is taken away than new bone is built. This makes your bones weak and more likely to break, which is why osteoporosis is often called "brittle bone disease." Osteoporosis has been called a silent disease because there are no outward signs or symptoms of the changes in bone density that are happening inside. In many cases, people become aware they have it only after a bone fracture. Considering that 40–50 percent of women in menopause will experience an osteoporotic fracture in their lifetimes, and the path to osteoporosis is long and can start in your thirties, the surprise diagnosis of osteoporosis likely happens far too often. This is why I want to make one point very clear: All women who are perimenopausal or menopausal should consider themselves at risk of developing osteoporosis and make building and supporting bone health a priority.

Strategies for Managing Your Risk of Osteoporosis

There are some general lifestyle strategies you can implement to help reduce your risk of osteoporosis, including not smoking (or stopping smoking) and limiting your intake of caffeine and alcohol. Both smoking and excessive alcohol and caffeine consumption have been found to decrease bone density and increase risk of fracture.

You can also take steps to reduce your risk of fracture by incorporating balance training exercises and removing tripping hazards from your environment. We tend to think of fall-proofing our homes as an activity reserved for individuals over the age of seventy, but trust me—with a cellphone in hand and four bags of groceries hanging off one arm as we bust through our front doors, we are all just as susceptible to an upturned rug corner or protruding table leg. A quick scan and some subtle shifts in placement can make all the difference when you're distracted.

And please, if you have that thing in your house that you've narrowly missed tripping on several times, every time thinking, "I really should move that!"—GO RIGHT NOW AND MOVE IT. No matter your age or menopausal status, recovering from a fall is no picnic (and recovery is obviously much longer and tougher if the fall results in a fracture); there's no downside to implementing this fall-prevention strategy.

NUTRITION

Pay attention to your protein intake: Protein is essential for muscle tissue maintenance, and muscle is crucial to helping protect your bones. See sidebar on page 237 for specific protein intake recommendations.

Get calcium from foods: Along with vitamin D, calcium is essential to the formation of bone tissue, and you want to ensure you are getting enough into your body to support strong bones. Ideally, you will get most of your calcium from foods, as some research suggests that high intake of supplemental calcium may increase risk of kidney stones and coronary artery disease. Some of the best food sources of calcium include:

- canned sardines and salmon (with bones—don't worry, they are soft and edible)

- dairy foods, such as ricotta, yogurt, and milk

- dark leafy greens, such as collard greens, broccoli rabe, kale, bok choy

- soybeans

SUPPLEMENTATION

You might need to take supplemental calcium to help you achieve the recommended daily intake of 1,000–1,200 mg/day, but again I strongly suggest that you meet most of this need with food. As I mentioned above, the use of supplemental calcium has been linked to increased risk of kidney stones and cardiovascular disease, the latter specifically in postmenopausal women. And higher doses of calcium supplementation have not been shown to be more bone protective.

Vitamin D is essential to helping your body absorb calcium. A minimum daily dose of 600 international units (IU) is recommended if you are between the ages of nineteen and fifty, and 800 IU if you are over fifty.

Creatine: Supplemental creatine (5g/day, usually in powder form) can help replenish the lower levels of creatine often seen in menopausal women, potentially resulting in improved muscle function and bone density. This supplement is especially beneficial when used in combination with resistance training, and it's also been found to help improve mood and cognition.

There is a lot of research to support the use of creatine for bone health, including one study showing that twelve months of creatine supplementation combined with resistance training resulted in increased bone mineral density in the femoral neck—which is not the neck that supports your head, but the "neck" or top of your femur near the hip joint. Bone density in the femoral neck is considered a predictor of fracture risk in postmenopausal women.

This same study found that creatine use also increased bone bending strength, which means that the bones developed a greater tolerance to stress—that is, it would take more for them to fracture.

Participants in this study took 0.1 gram of creatine per kilogram of body weight per day and completed three days a week of resistance training. A reasonable, safe, and effective dose is likely 5 g/day for most menopausal women.

Long-term use of specific *bioactive collagen peptides* (Fortibone) has been shown to help slow down the loss of bone mineral density in people with osteoporosis or osteopenia (low bone density that may precede osteoporosis). Maintaining bone mineral density can help reduce risk of fracture and other bone-related injuries. Participants in the study took 5 grams of Fortibone bioactive collagen peptides each day for four years. It is usually found in powder form and mixed with water.

EXERCISE

Resistance training places a load on bones, which when repeated can increase bone strength. *Weight-bearing exercises* such as dancing, walking, jogging, tai chi, hiking, and racquet sports like pickleball and tennis can also help strengthen bones and improve balance.

PHARMACOLOGIC OPTIONS

Menopausal hormone therapy has been shown in randomized controlled trials (including in the Women's Health Initiative) to reduce the risk of osteoporosis-related fractures. This risk reduction has been seen both in women who have established osteoporosis and in those who are at low risk of osteoporotic fracture.

For bone protection, a transdermal 50 microgram patch, oral estradiol of 2 milligrams, or conjugated equine estrogens at 0.625 milligram may be most effective, but lower doses can also be protective. (The transdermal estradiol patch is what I prefer for myself and my patients; see chapter 7 for more on MHT.)

Other medications for osteoporosis work by helping to control the way your bones break down and build up, which increases bone strength. Depending on what you need, your doctor might suggest medicines that can help slow the breakdown of your bones. These can include things like estrogen receptor (ER) agonists, bisphosphonates, or a medicine called denosumab, which helps to stop the process that breaks down bones.

Pain with Intercourse, see Sexual Dysfunction

Palpitations, see Heart Palpitations

Sarcopenia

Sarcopenia is a progressive age-related condition characterized by the loss of skeletal muscle mass, strength, and function. It often leads to reduced physical performance and an increased risk of falls and fractures, which obviously affects your overall quality of life. Research has found that hormonal fluctuations during menopause can lead to sarcopenia and influence muscle loss earlier than we might expect; a change in muscle mass has been noted between the early and late stages of perimenopause.

As I mentioned in chapter 6, estrogen and testosterone play an important role in the maintenance of muscle tissue. When these levels decline, we begin to lose muscle, often without even realizing it. The loss of muscle mass can in turn contribute to bone density reduction, potentially leading to conditions like osteoporosis. Muscle and bone health are strongly tied to one another metabolically and anatomically and often mirror one another in either strength or weakness. For this reason, you'll notice that many of the strategies in each area overlap.

It's critical to take steps to maintain muscle mass (and there's no such thing as focusing too soon on muscle preservation). After all, muscle mass plays a crucial role in maintaining your overall health; it is involved in so many aspects of physical capabilities, metabolism, and well-being, including:

- FRAILTY PREVENTION: Maintaining muscle mass is vital in preventing frailty, especially in older women. Frailty is a syndrome characterized by a decline in physical function and a heightened vulnerability to adverse health outcomes. Loss of muscle mass is a primary contributor to frailty, leading to weakness, reduced mobility, and an increased risk of falls and fractures.

- PHYSICAL FUNCTION: Strong muscles provide the strength and endurance needed for everyday activities, from climbing stairs and carrying groceries to maintaining balance and preventing injuries. In women, particularly older women, preserving muscle mass is essential for maintaining independence and a high quality of life.

- INSULIN SENSITIVITY AND GLUCOSE CONTROL: Muscle tissue plays a significant role in glucose metabolism. Skeletal muscles are responsible for taking up and utilizing glucose from the bloodstream, making muscle tissue an essential ally in protecting insulin sensitivity. This is crucial in preventing or managing conditions like type 2 diabetes and insulin resistance, to which we become more susceptible during menopause.

- BASAL METABOLIC RATE (BMR): Muscle tissue is metabolically active, meaning it burns calories even at rest. Having more muscle increases your basal metabolic rate (BMR), which is the number of calories your body needs to maintain basic physiological functions like breathing, circulation, and cell repair. Women with higher muscle mass tend to have a higher BMR, making it easier to maintain a healthy weight and manage body composition.

- BONE HEALTH: While muscle and bone are distinct tissues, they are closely interconnected. Resistance exercises that build and maintain muscle also put stress on bones, leading to increased bone density. This is so important for us as we age! Maintaining robust bone density can protect against injury and fracture.

- WEIGHT MANAGEMENT: Muscle mass can aid in weight management and body composition. Muscle tissue is denser than fat tissue, which means that having more muscle can make you not just stronger but leaner as well. Plus, the higher BMR associated with increased muscle mass will burn additional calories.

The diagnosis of sarcopenia typically involves assessing muscle mass with a dual-energy X-ray absorptiometry (DEXA) scanner or an InBody scanner and testing strength. I have an InBody scanner that I use for measuring my patients' muscle mass. I also have a detailed discussion with all my patients about muscle mass and the many ways it can affect health. My overall plan for symptom improvement often leans heavily on strategies that will protect and build muscle tissue.

Strategies for Coping with Sarcopenia

Treating and preventing sarcopenia require the combination of high-quality nutrition and physical activity to enhance muscle strength and physical performance. Also, because inflammation may play a role in advancing the breakdown of muscle tissue, eating plenty of anti-inflammatory foods, minimizing alcohol consumption, not smoking, getting adequate sleep, and implementing stress reduction practices will help you protect valuable muscle tissue.

NUTRITION

Studies have shown that beneficial nutrition strategies include an increased intake of fruits and vegetables; a recommended minimum daily intake of 1.2 grams or more of protein per kilogram of body weight; and the ingestion of a high-protein meal or shake containing 20 grams of protein soon after exercise to support muscle tissue maintenance and development.

In addition to dietary protein, it's important to make sure you are getting enough vitamin D and calcium, which are essential to supporting bone health. Osteoporosis and sarcopenia are interconnected through their impact on musculoskeletal health and overall physical function. Adequate calcium and vitamin D are crucial in addressing and preventing both conditions. Calcium supports bone health, and vitamin D aids in calcium absorption while also playing a role in muscle function. If you are at risk of or dealing with osteoporosis and sarcopenia, it's important to consult with healthcare professionals to assess your specific nutritional needs and to develop a personalized plan for maintaining musculoskeletal health and preventing fractures and muscle weakness.

EXERCISE

The most effective exercise regimen in treating sarcopenia appears to be one that combines aerobic exercise and resistance training. A consistent commitment to resistance training is invaluable in preventing sarcopenia, as it has been shown to help build and preserve muscle mass and strength. A Cochrane review (conducted and published by the Cochrane Collaboration, a trusted group of medical experts) suggests that progressive resistance training two to three times per week is particularly beneficial.

I have made a personal commitment to make muscle growth and maintenance a high priority for myself, which is why my goal is to get at least three strength workouts a week. If you'd like more guidance in this area, an excellent resource is the book *Forever Strong* by Dr. Gabrielle Lyon.

It's important to point out that while resistance training is ideal for developing and maintaining muscle tissue, if for whatever reason you can't commit to it, do something else; find the exercise that you can make a consistent commitment to and keep doing it. Regular physical activity helps protect against many diseases; increases mood, energy, and self-esteem; benefits metabolism; strengthens your heart . . . the list goes on and on. Exercise really is the best medicine.

SUPPLEMENTATION

Studies show that postmenopausal women who take *creatine* supplements (5 g/day) while doing strength training exercises can increase their muscle mass and strength.

Selenium, magnesium, and omega-3 fatty acids may help preserve muscle mass and protect muscle tissue from inflammatory damage.

PHARMACOLOGIC OPTIONS

Menopausal hormone therapy (MHT) has shown mixed results in preserving muscle mass in postmenopausal women. While it may benefit muscle power and what we call contraction regulation, its impact on muscle mass remains uncertain (although testosterone therapy has been shown to improve muscle tone and mass in menopausal women).

How Much Protein Is Enough?

It's crucial to increase your protein intake during menopause to support your overall health and to specifically protect and preserve muscle mass and function. As women age, our protein requirements tend to increase because of several factors, including changes in muscle protein synthesis and the increased risk of muscle loss that comes with hormone changes. If you become insulin resistant, which as you may recall you are at a greater risk of in menopause, you may need a higher protein intake to maintain muscle mass and function. This is because insulin resistance can impair your body's ability to use dietary protein effectively for muscle protein synthesis.

Several observational studies have highlighted the positive association between higher protein intake and better muscle health in postmenopausal women. For example, research from the Women's Health Initiative found that a protein intake of 1.2 grams per kilogram of body weight was linked to a 32 percent lower risk of frailty and better physical function. An even greater intake of 1.6 grams per kilogram of body weight was associated with higher skeletal muscle mass index in postmenopausal women. (To run this calculation, you may need to find an online calculator to convert your weight in pounds to your weight in kilograms. Once you have this latter number, multiply it by either 1.2 or 1.6 grams to get your ideal protein intake in grams.)

It should be noted that this level of protein intake is higher than the general recommended daily allowance (RDA) of protein, which is 0.8 gram per kilogram of body weight. But based on what we know about postmenopausal risk for muscle loss and frailty, I feel strongly that this RDA is simply not enough protein and you should instead aim for at least between 1.2 to 1.6 grams per kilogram of body weight.

When you are looking to increase your protein intake, be sure to eat a variety of sources, including lean meats, poultry, fish, dairy, legumes, and plant-based options. Doing so will help ensure that you're getting all the essential nutrients and amino acids necessary for muscle maintenance and overall health. Also, as you pay more attention to your protein intake, pay attention to when you eat it as well—it's best to divide protein between your snacks and meals throughout the day rather than eating it all in one sitting.

Sexual Dysfunction

I'm sixty years old. I have been struggling through menopause for ten years. First, itchy patches of skin that felt like electric shocks under my skin, mood swings, rage, headaches, flu-like feeling once a month, exhaustion, hot flashes, night sweats, loss of self-confidence, brain fog, no sex drive, vaginal dryness, horrible pain during sex, weight gain, nonexistent orgasms, depression. My sex life is abysmal. My husband has been so patient, so loving, and even so creative in bed, but things I used to love the feel of, sexually, I feel no more. I'm not turned off by them, I just feel nothing physically. The hardest symptom I continue to have that brings me to my knees is—prior to a hot flash, I get the saddest feeling I've ever experienced. It's a feeling of utter darkness. It lasts a split second then I break out into a sweat. Then the feeling disappears. After a full day of this happening fifteen-plus times, I am emotionally exhausted and questioning everything in my life. I feel so broken.

—Elizabeth L.

Sexual function is a complex and integral part of overall well-being and quality of life. During menopause, it's common to experience changes in your sexual health, which can be distressing and have a significant impact on your relationships. Understanding the causes of sexual dysfunction during menopause can help remove the mystery around any changes you've experienced, and exploring treatment options can give you hope that relief (and a return to sexual pleasure) are both on the horizon.

Sexual dysfunction in menopause can manifest in a few ways, such as:

- HYPOACTIVE SEXUAL DESIRE DISORDER (HSDD): HSDD is characterized by a persistent or recurrent lack of sexual fantasies and desire for sexual activity. The prevalence of HSDD is higher in midlife women, ranging from 14.5 to 33 percent, and may occur because of hormonal changes, psychological factors, and relationship issues. I estimate that nearly 50 percent of the patients I see in my menopause-focused clinic have HSDD.

- AROUSAL DISORDER: It's common in menopause to feel difficulties around sexual arousal, and it's not just in your head. Reduced sexual arousal happens as a result of reduced genital blood flow, vaginal dryness, and decreased sensitivity. These physical changes can lead to discomfort during sexual activity and reduced sexual desire.

- ORGASMIC DISORDER: Hormonal changes, decreased blood flow to the pelvic region, or psychological factors can lead to difficulty reaching orgasm or create less intense orgasms during menopause.

- PAIN DURING SEX: Genitourinary syndrome of menopause (GSM) can lead to painful sexual intercourse. The thinning and drying of vaginal tissues can cause discomfort, burning, or pain during sex, leading to a decline in sexual desire. (See also the GSM entry on page 192.)

- RELATIONSHIP ISSUES: Changes in sexual desire and function can strain intimate relationships. Even if you feel connected and supported by a partner, a lack of desire or interest in physical intimacy can lead to disconnection and distance.

242 THE NEW MENOPAUSE

Strategies for Dealing with Sexual Dysfunction

As a physician who works with women, I feel it's crucial for me to initiate discussions about sexual health during menopause and offer a safe space for my patients to express their concerns. Too many women struggle with changes to their sexual health—and they don't need to. Your doctor can work with you to create a personalized treatment plan that considers the specific factors contributing to your experience with sexual dysfunction. You can regain sexual satisfaction and improve your overall quality of life in menopause, but it all starts with you being willing to be open about your symptoms with your doctor or healthcare practitioner.

In my clinic, I have all my patients complete this checklist. You can also complete it to help give you talking points to discuss with your doctor.

Sexual Symptom Checklist

Please answer these questions about your overall sexual function in the past three months.

1. Are you satisfied with your sexual function?
   Yes/No. If No, please continue.

2. How long have you been dissatisfied with your sexual function?

   _____

3. The problem(s) with your sexual function is (mark one or more)

   a. Problem with little or no interest in sex

   b. Problem with decreased genital sensation (feeling)

   c. Problem with decreased vaginal lubrication (dryness)

   d. Problem reaching orgasm

   e. Problem with pain during sex

   f. Other _____

4. Which problem (in question 3) is most bothersome?
   (Circle a, b, c, d, e, or f)

5. Would you like to talk about it with your healthcare provider?
   Yes/No

Leading a healthy lifestyle that includes anti-inflammatory nutrition, regular exercise, and stress-reduction practices can enhance overall well-being and sexual function. In a lot of cases, though, addressing sexual dysfunction during menopause will require more than just lifestyle adjustments. A comprehensive approach that considers physical, psychological, and relational aspects is often the most effective.

Nonpharmacological treatment options include:

- EDUCATION: Educating yourself about menopausal changes, sexual health, and expectations can help you better understand your body and alleviate concerns. A great reference in this area is Dr. Kelly Casperson's book (and podcast of the same name) *You Are Not Broken*. I also recommend *Come As You Are* by Emily Nagowski.

- PSYCHOTHERAPY: Individual or couples' therapy, such as cognitive-behavioral therapy or sex therapy, can help address psychological issues, improve communication, and enhance intimacy.

- PELVIC FLOOR THERAPY: For women with pelvic floor issues contributing to sexual dysfunction, physical therapy can be beneficial.

- ALTERNATIVE THERAPIES: Some women find relief from sexual dysfunction symptoms through complementary therapies such as acupuncture or mindfulness practices.

- COMMUNICATION: Open and honest communication with a partner is vital for addressing relationship issues related to sexual dysfunction. Couples' counseling can facilitate discussions and solutions.

Pharmacologic options include:

- HORMONE THERAPY: Hormone therapy, including estrogen and testosterone replacement, can address the genitourinary symptoms of menopause that contribute to sexual dysfunction. Testosterone therapy, in particular, has shown great promise in improving sexual desire in menopausal women. See page 101 for more information.

- FDA-APPROVED MEDICATIONS: There are two medications that are FDA approved for the treatment of sexual desire disorders in premenopausal women. They are used frequently off-label for postmenopausal women, but the testing was done in premenopausal women. These medications are *flibanserin*, which enhances sexual desire by affecting serotonin receptors,and *bremelanotide*, which acts on melanocortin receptors to increase sexual desire.

- VAGINAL MOISTURIZERS AND LUBRICANTS: Over-the-counter or prescription vaginal moisturizers and lubricants can alleviate vaginal dryness and discomfort during sex.

Skin Changes

I didn't realize my body was experiencing perimenopause symptoms at thirty-eight. I felt like aliens had taken my real body and replaced it with an imposter. A foreign body with anxiety, memory loss, dry skin, itchy skin, hot flashes, irritability, irregular periods, and that was just the beginning! I truly felt lost, alone, and if I'm being honest, completely crazy! My mom passed away at sixty-two, and I was the first of my girlfriends to go through the "change." I felt alone and didn't have anyone to talk to. I was white-knuckling it through this phase and simply wanted to feel like my old happy, noncrazy self. My best friend told me to follow Dr. Haver on social media. Dr. Haver gave me tools to help me help myself. Forever grateful!

—Jennifer H.

There's no denying that your skin will change during menopause. This is largely due to the fact that menopause brings on an accelerated loss of collagen, elastin, and water in the skin, a trifecta that can lead to several skin changes, including increased skin sensitivity. The decline in estrogen that begins in perimenopause also causes less blood flow to your skin, resulting in poorer wound repair, and can contribute to a decrease in facial fat, which can alter the contours of your face. Other skin changes that may occur around menopause include:

- dry skin

- wrinkles/collagen loss

- impaired wound healing/barrier function

- thinning skin

- itchy skin

- itchy ears (the skin of the ears seems especially susceptible to these changes, and it's a harder area to treat)

- eczema

- dermatitis

- increased perception of aging

The changes in collagen, elastin, and water that occur in menopause can contribute in their own ways to the changes we may see in the mirror.

Collagen is a protein present in the skin that is responsible for its strength and elasticity. We lose nearly a *third of our skin collagen* in the first five years after menopause and will continue to lose an additional 2 percent each year during the next fifteen years. This collagen loss occurs postmenopause, independent of chronological age.

Elastin is a protein that is responsible for the elasticity of the skin. When we lose elastin in menopause, the result is increased wrinkling and a noticeable slack in skin.

Water loss plays an important role in how effective your skin is as a barrier and helps prevent skin dryness. During our premenopausal years, our skin cells retain water as a way to boost resilience to external irritants and to maintain moisture. However, during menopause we start to experience what's referred to as transepidermal water loss (TEWL), which diminishes the integrity of our skin barrier and contributes to dryness. Both of these changes lead to more sensitive skin that's prone to pruritus (itching), xerosis (extremely dry skin), eczema, and dermatitis. Unfortunately, simply drinking more water does not offset this biological water loss.

Strategies for Addressing Skin Changes

As your largest organ, your skin responds to the same practices of good health that will bring out the best in the rest of your body. These include eating an anti-inflammatory diet rich in antioxidants that help protect against cellular damage; exercising to increase blood circulation; and not drinking alcohol excessively or smoking.

It's also essential to protect your skin from the sun's UV rays, which cause skin damage that advances aging and puts you at increased risk of skin cancer. Proper UV protection strategies include:

- using the most effective sunscreens available, which are currently those that contain zinc or titanium oxide. Effective sunscreen use also includes reapplying as often as a brand's directions recommend.

- wearing UV protective clothing

- avoiding peak sunlight hours

In addition to these baseline skin health and protection practices, there are some other strategies that may help improve your skin in menopause.

PHARMACOLOGIC OPTIONS

Systemic estrogen therapy has been shown to reduce transepidermal water loss, which may help reduce occurrences of dermatitis and other skin conditions. Estrogen therapy has also been shown to increase skin collagen levels to premenopausal states and to help increase skin thickness and prevent further collagen loss. Results can be seen as early as three months after beginning MHT, and the increase in collagen seems to happen regardless of how estrogen is delivered to your system.

Some studies have shown that topical estrogen can increase elastin when applied to areas such as the buttocks and abdomen. I am using a topical estriol cream (by prescription) and recommending it to my patients. However, systemic estrogen (96) did not help increase elastin levels.

There's also a developing market of skin care products containing phytoestrogens and selective estrogen receptor modulators (SERMs), which are capable of directly addressing estrogen deficiency in the skin. They are showing promise, but at the time of this publication there is not enough research for me to recommend these options over other treatments.

PRODUCTS/TREATMENTS

Several products can help improve skin health as your hormones change during the menopausal transition and beyond. I've listed some of them here. I also suggest following Dr. Anthony Youn on social media for the most current developments in the area of skin health and protection.

- Moisturizers with ingredients like ceramides and hyaluronic acid can help retain moisture and hydration in the skin.

- The use of 4'-acetoxy resveratrol (4AR) and equol has been shown in studies to help improve skin health and appearance in menopause. Available over the counter.

- Other research has shown that oral intake of a collagen peptide called Verisol increased levels of elastin and a key precursor to collagen and produced significant reduction in eye wrinkles. (This is the collagen I use in the formula for my 'Pause Life collagen supplement; I've used it for years!)

- Topical retinoids and alpha- and beta-hydroxy acids can improve skin texture.

- Peels, fractional lasers, vascular-specific lasers, and intense pulsed-light treatments offered by your dermatologist or a medispa can target specific skin goals.

- Hyaluronic acid fillers and toxins like botulinum toxin (Botox) injections can temporarily address wrinkles and volume loss.

- Radiofrequency and focused ultrasound treatments stimulate collagen production and tissue remodeling in deeper skin layers.

- Collagen stimulators, like poly-L-lactic acid, restore underlying skin structure, and modified hyaluronic acids can provide volume and lift in specific facial areas.

Sleep Apnea

> I have no get up 'n' go, I have the spare tire, the back fat, armpit fat, brain fog, sleep apnea, mouth breather, and depression. These symptoms gradually started in my early forties, and now I'm almost fifty-three and still in perimenopause. I'm frustrated and I just want to feel better!
>
> —Tami F.

Obstructive sleep apnea (OSA) is a potentially serious breathing disorder that can block your upper airway during sleep and cause you to struggle to breathe or stop breathing altogether. It's linked to increased risk of cardiovascular disease, stroke, metabolic disorders, and a decline in neurocognitive functions related to learning, memory, and language.

OSA has been traditionally associated with men, but recent research has revealed a link between menopause and obstructive sleep apnea. The findings determined that decreasing estrogen during menopause can affect upper airway muscles and increase the chances of airway collapse during sleep. The research in this area is relatively new and developing, so what we know about the relationship between menopause and OSA may change over time. However, it's critical that we raise awareness that the association between sleep apnea and menopausal women exists. There is a clear gender gap in OSA diagnosis and treatment, perhaps because women don't demonstrate the same symptoms as men. Rather than loud snoring or gasping for air during sleep, women are more likely to experience daytime sleepiness, which practitioners may blame on other factors, such as depression or ... well, menopause. And women who do snore (having been told so by a bedside companion) may feel an embarrassment about reporting the symptom, especially if it's been noted as being loud.

The truth is that it's dangerous to be quiet about symptoms of sleep apnea, given its link to significant health risks. If you experience chronic daytime sleepiness, mood changes, daytime cognitive issues such as trouble concentrating, or repeated wake-ups throughout the night, or if you've been told you snore or have strange pauses in breathing during your sleep, you should consider being evaluated for sleep apnea.

Strategies for Dealing with Sleep Apnea

Risk factors for sleep apnea include overweight or obesity, smoking, alcohol use, hypertension, type 2 diabetes, and hyperlipidemia (high cholesterol). In menopause, the loss of muscle and the increase in abdominal obesity can also combine to create increased risk of OSA. You can therefore potentially reduce your risk for and symptoms of sleep apnea by focusing on the same lifestyle modifications that can support your overall health during menopause. These include eating an anti-inflammatory diet and getting regular exercise.

Hopefully, increased research into the link between menopause and sleep apnea will soon lead to an expanded list of ways to treat this potentially serious breathing disorder.

PHARMACOLOGIC OPTIONS

A continuous positive airway pressure (CPAP) machine is a device that you wear while sleeping that delivers air into your airway to help prevent blockages. It can be tough to be consistent with CPAP use, but it's a very effective way to reduce sleep apnea and the related risks and symptoms.

Oral appliances, mouthpieces that push the lower jaw and tongue forward, can sometimes help treat OSA. You can get these from a dental health provider.

Research from the mid-2000s found that *hormone replacement therapy (MHT)* may reduce the severity of sleep-disordered breathing in women going through menopause. Again, we need more research in this area!

Sleep Disturbances

> I am 48. I started with drenching night sweats and insomnia 1.5 years ago. Then, heart palpitations, dry skin, painful sex, zero libido, and my hair stopped growing. My doctor ran my FSH and it was normal, and said, "Nope, not menopause. Try this Celexa." I felt worse. I tried a six-month trial of Maca and other supplements and saw no improvement. I had joint aches, no energy, fatigue, and an increase in belly fat. I had at least fifty hot flashes per day. I finally had enough and told the doctor that I wanted hormone therapy. After two weeks of taking estradiol and progesterone, I had no hot flashes, I was sleeping well, and my palpitations were gone. I can't believe I didn't do it sooner; I'm now looking forward to the future.
>
> —Sheri D.

Sleep problems often become more prevalent and noticeable during the menopausal transition because of several factors, including natural aging; psychological issues, such as increased occurrence of anxiety and depression; coexisting health conditions that may disrupt sleep, such as obstructive sleep apnea (OSA); and symptoms of menopause, such as night sweats. These factors can independently or collectively lead to insomnia, which is an established destroyer of quality of life and one of the most common sleep disorders reported among menopausal women. According to the American Psychiatric Association, insomnia disorder is defined as experiencing a sleep complaint that occurs at least three times per week for at least three months and is associated with distress or impaired daytime functioning. A sleep complaint might be something like difficulty falling asleep, nonrestorative sleep, and difficulty staying asleep.

A study using data from the National Health Interview Survey found that sleep complaints tend to vary based on your menopausal stage: Peri-menopausal women were more likely to sleep less than seven hours per night and report poor sleep quality, and postmenopausal women were more likely to have trouble falling asleep and staying asleep.

The four major categories of possible causes of insomnia in menopausal women are:

1. *Menopause-related insomnia:* Often related to vasomotor symptoms like hot flashes and night sweats, this type of insomnia is commonly underdiagnosed or misdiagnosed.

2. *Primary insomnia:* This is psychophysiological and can be related to factors such as anxiety and poor sleep habits.

3. *Secondary insomnia:* This is associated with underlying sleep disorders, mental or medical conditions, or aging.

4. *Insomnia induced by behavioral, environmental, or psychosocial factors:* These factors can include lifestyle choices, stress, and environmental conditions.

STRATEGIES FOR DEALING WITH SLEEP DISTURBANCES

In most cases, improving your sleep quality and duration requires a multifaceted approach that considers potential underlying causes. One good place to start is to work on improving your sleep hygiene by creating a consistent sleep schedule, ensuring that your sleep environment is comfortable (the right temperature, no disruptive lighting, a comfortable pillow), and eliminating your exposure to blue light–emitting devices (cellphone, tablet, LED TV screens) two or more hours prior to bedtime. I know this last one sounds difficult, but as an experiment try swapping out a TV show or constant scrolling for a board game, a physical book, or conversation before bed to see if you notice any improvements.

THERAPEUTIC OPTIONS

There are also different types of therapy that may help improve your sleep. For each of the therapeutic options, it is best to seek out the help of a sleep medicine specialist or sleep therapist. These include:

- COGNITIVE BEHAVIORAL THERAPY FOR INSOMNIA (CBT-I): This type of talk therapy can help identify and change negative thoughts and behaviors that may be contributing to your sleep problems.

- STIMULUS-CONTROL THERAPY: This technique focuses on creating a strong association between your bed and sleep by limiting activities in bed to sleep and sex.

- RELAXATION THERAPY: Techniques like progressive muscle relaxation and deep breathing exercises can help reduce anxiety and promote relaxation before bedtime.

- SLEEP-RESTRICTION THERAPY: This approach involves limiting the time spent in bed to increase sleep efficiency and consolidate sleep.

SUPPLEMENTATION

Some women have reported improved sleep with the use of magnesium supplementation, particularly in the form of magnesium L-threonate. This type of magnesium has been associated with better sleep quality and reduced "racing thoughts" at night. However, remember that supplements are not regulated, and product quality and purity can vary.

PHARMACOLOGIC OPTIONS

Some pharmacologic treatments for sleep disturbances can be effective, but be sure to discuss the potential side effects and contraindications with your doctor, and always use them under the guidance of a healthcare provider.

Many of the medications used to improve sleep during menopause target the improvement of hot flashes since these are so disruptive to sleep. These include:

- MENOPAUSAL HORMONE THERAPY (MHT): while not indicated for the treatment of primary sleep disorders, MHT is effective at reducing nighttime vasomotor symptoms

- SELECTIVE SEROTONIN REUPTAKE INHIBITORS (SSRIS): escitalopram and paroxetine

- SEROTONIN-NOREPINEPHRINE REUPTAKE INHIBITORS (SNRIS): venlafaxine

- GABA AGENTS: gabapentin

Other pharmacological treatments may approach different aspects of sleep disturbances:

- MELATONIN RECEPTOR AGONISTS: Ramelteon is a melatonin receptor agonist and may be prescribed to help address sleep-onset difficulties.

- OREXIN RECEPTOR ANTAGONISTS: Suvorexant is a new medication that reduces arousal and wakefulness, potentially helping with insomnia characterized by difficulty falling asleep.

Temporomandibular Disorder

In perimenopause, I began suffering greatly from TMJ. I also started noticing ringing in my ears, and neither have ever stopped. I wear a small mouth guard at night to help with TMJ in case I clench my jaw, but it does not seem to help. I have had it for about eight years now. Ringing in my ears is 24/7/365. It never ever goes away, but sometimes it's super loud.

—Maureen D.

You have two joints called the temporomandibular joints (TMJ) that together connect the lower jaw to the skull and allow for the jaw movements involved in eating, talking, and more. In temporomandibular disorder (TMD), the joints, muscles, bones, and nerves involved in these movements can become irritated and can cause significant pain, head-aches, toothaches, and difficulty talking. TMD can also result from a dis-located jaw or bone loss in the jaw. Women are *three times more likely* than men to develop chronic TMD, which is defined as experiencing jaw pain for at least six months.

The fact that so many more women than men experience TMD has led researchers to investigate a hormonal link. Studies have shown that inci-dence of TMD peaks between the ages of forty-five and sixty-four, which coincides with the decreasing hormone levels associated with menopause. It's well established that the loss of estrogen can lead to an increase in in-flammatory proteins, such as cytokines, which initiate and contribute to the progression of disorders of the temporomandibular joints. Additional research that compared the prevalence and severity of TMD between menopausal and premenopausal women found that TMD was signifi-cantly more common in menopausal women.

Strategies for Managing TMD

If you have TMD symptoms, such as frequent headaches, toothaches, dif-ficulty talking, or painful clicking or popping in the jaw, you will want to see your dentist for treatment options. A wide variety of strategies may be suggested, including anti-inflammatory medications such as ibuprofen, Botox injections, muscle relaxants, topical ointments, and acupuncture.

PHARMACOLOGIC OPTIONS

Menopause hormone therapy (MHT) has been shown to have a modest impact on the progression of TMD, meaning it may help slow the develop-ment of the disorder. Given what we know about the role hormone replacement can play in helping restore bone density, MHT may be espe-cially helpful in TMD that's caused by loss of bone in the jaw.

Researchers are also exploring the different estrogen signaling path-ways that may be involved in controlling pain in temporomandibular dis-orders. Selective estrogen receptor modulators (SERMs), which are medications that bind to estrogen receptors to help turn them "on" or "off," may be a potentially effective pharmacologic treatment in TMD.

Thinning Hair (on Head), see Androgen-Induced Conditions

Thinning Skin, see Skin Changes

Tingling Extremities, see Crawling Skin Sensations

Tinnitus

I'm a fifty-five-year-old woman, mom of twin nineteen-year-olds, ideal body weight and in good health. I'm a registered dietitian, eat healthy, and exercise as part of my daily life plan. I would say I was officially in menopause at approximately fifty-one years old. My main complaint symptoms of menopause were hot flashes! Definitely severe. My gynecologist asked if I experienced more than five per day and that was laughable! I would have too many to count. I suffered for a couple years with hot flashes and other symptoms. I thought I could manage it with my healthy lifestyle. What a mistake! Wasted time! Eventually I went to a menopause gynecologist and started on an estradiol patch and progesterone with great results!

My other menopause symptoms I figured out later were vertigo and tinnitus! although at the time, I did not put this together and neither did my doctors. I even scheduled an appointment with an ENT. He never factored menopause as a contributor to my problems. He felt my tinnitus was due to a concert I attended sitting in the front row. My vertigo was never explained. However, later that year, I started HRT and these symptoms were greatly minimized! I'm glad to be on the other side now!

—Debbi H.

Tinnitus is an auditory condition that creates the sensation of a ringing, buzzing, or hissing sound in the ears. This phantom noise can range from mildly bothersome to profoundly distressing, affecting an individual's quality of life. While tinnitus can result from various factors such as hearing loss, loud noise exposure, medications, and psychological stress, recent research has hinted at a potential link between tinnitus and menopause and revealed that *22 percent* of postmenopausal women have reportedly experienced tinnitus.

Several studies have suggested that reproductive hormones may play a role in the development of tinnitus. This isn't entirely surprising, as low estrogen levels in menopause have been linked to hearing loss, so we know it plays a role in auditory function. Estrogen influences blood flow into the ear and reduces cochlear inflammation and damage to neurons essential to auditory pathways. When estrogen declines in menopause, issues such as tinnitus and hearing loss become more common. Unfortunately, we need more research before we can describe estrogen's precise contribution to these auditory changes.

Strategies for Dealing with Tinnitus

Tinnitus can be an incredibly bothersome and disruptive condition. I hope with time we understand more about the relationship between tinnitus and menopause so that more targeted and effective treatments can be developed. If you are dealing with tinnitus during menopause, be sure to discuss with your doctor or see an audiologist for additional treatments or protocols that may provide relief.

PHARMACOLOGIC OPTIONS

In one study, *menopausal hormone therapy (MHT)* users were found to have a *50.5 percent lower risk of developing tinnitus compared to nonusers.* This result suggests that MHT may have benefits in managing and preventing tinnitus, but we need more evidence to confirm its effectiveness.

TMJ, see Temporomandibular Disorder

Unwanted Hair Growth (Whiskers), see Androgen-Induced Conditions

Urinary Tract Infections, see Genitourinary Syndrome

Vaginal Dryness, see Genitourinary Syndrome

Vertigo

I am fifty-two years old, and cruising along, managing just fine. My periods have been erratic since 2018 when I began to experience extreme hair loss and anxiety about everything, terrible sleep, and extreme fatigue. My patience was also much shorter at this time. Fast forward to 2022, and along with the hair loss, anxiety, and weight gain (despite a better diet), lack of sleep, why not add in some heart palpitations just for fun? Due to my own ignorance about Peri/Meno at this time, a trip to the ER, and wearing a monitor for seventy-two hours, the doctor told me I was fine and offered zero explanation. In August 2022, I had a twelve-day period and noticed the start of hot/cold flashes, and they were coming fast and furious. In September 2023, I was hit with vertigo and was still suffering with dizziness daily. I read and implemented the Galveston Diet, and the hot/cold flashes subsided and my sleep was so much better, but dizziness continues.

—Alayna H.

Vertigo, including benign paroxysmal positional vertigo (BPPV), presents as sudden episodes of dizziness or spinning sensations, often triggered by specific head movements. These episodes can be disorienting and distressing, affecting a person's balance and spatial orientation. The prevalence of BPPV is notably higher in women than in men, and clinical experience suggests that menopause may be a contributing factor. This is due to the fact that hormonal fluctuations can influence the inner ear, which is responsible for maintaining balance and spatial orientation. Menopause may also lead to vertigo by affecting:

- OTOCONIA DISLODGMENT: Within the inner ear, tiny calcium crystals known as otoconia play a crucial role in balance. During menopause, hormonal fluctuations can affect the inner ear's stability, leading to the dislodgment of these calcium crystals and triggering BPPV.

- OTOCONIA METABOLISM: The decrease in estrogen levels during menopause can impair the metabolism of otoconia and lead to fewer of these calcium crystals that are essential to your sense of balance and orientation.

- VISCOSITY AND VOLUME OF INNER EAR FLUID: Menopause-related hormonal changes can alter the viscosity and volume of the fluid within the inner ear. These changes can disrupt the delicate balance mechanisms, further contributing to vertigo symptoms.

Since not all women experience BPPV during menopause, it's clear that it's not hormone changes alone that cause it to develop. Age, genetics, and lifestyle can also influence the development of vertigo. Recent research has also suggested that there may be a connection between BPPV and bone density. Patients with BPPV, both women and men, have been found to exhibit lower bone density compared to controls. It's not clear yet what the connection is between the two, but the link raises concerns about the potential impact of BPPV on bone health. It also makes it clear that in patients with vertigo, bone density should be carefully and regularly monitored.

Strategies for Dealing with Vertigo

Studies have shown that reduced levels of *vitamin D* may contribute to the occurrence of BPPV. Supplementation of vitamin D, either alone or in combination with calcium, has been found to reduce recurrent episodes in BPPV patients.

Menopausal hormone therapy (MHT) was found to be better than placebo in decreasing the incidence of vertigo in menopausal women. This could be because replacing estrogen likely aids in the correction of otoconia metabolism, restoring the number of otoconia needed in the inner ear for stability and balance.

Combining hormone replacement and vitamin D management may be a more effective strategy for preventing recurrent vertigo attacks in perimenopausal women with BPPV.

The Epley maneuver is the most well-known version of canalith repositioning, a treatment used to help people with BPPV. It involves making specific head movements to relieve the dizzy feelings. This maneuver is like a trick to help put the tiny calcium particles inside your ear that have become dislodged back where they belong, which helps restore orientation and reduce the sensation of dizziness. It should be noted that this method doesn't work for other kinds of dizziness. Ask your doctor if you are a candidate for performing this procedure.

Weight Gain, see Body Composition Changes/Belly Fat

Wrinkles, see Skin Changes

My great hope is that the Tool Kit has been helpful to you and that you will share this resource with others. In the future, we expect to add more symptoms and solutions as our knowledge and understanding of menopause expands. You can be a part of this expansion by having open conversations about your own experience—and together we can continue to normalize and destigmatize menopause.

Helpful Menopause Resources

As I've mentioned several times, I maintain a "recommended physician registry" on my website. If you have a confirmed and awesome provider of quality menopausal care, I hope you will consider visiting thepauselife.com, where you can recommend your doctor's practice to our unbiased referral program. This way, others in your area who may be looking for a provider will discover the recommendation.

The Galveston Diet: galvestondiet.com

The 'Pause Life: thepauselife.com

Evernow: start.evernow.com

Alloy Health: myalloy.com

The Menopause Society: www.menopause.org

Midi Health: joinmidi.com

Updated Statements and Stats on the Use of Menopausal Hormone Therapy

You may find it helpful to bring the following recent, formal statements about the use of menopausal hormone therapy to your next doctor's appointment. Offer it in the spirit of collaboration, perhaps by saying, "Here's some info from credible sources on the use of hormone therapy in menopausal women. I hope we can work together to determine the most appropriate course of treatment for my symptoms."

In 2022, **the North American Menopause Society (NAMS)**, now the Menopause Society, issued an updated position on hormone therapy, "The 2022 Hormone Therapy Position Statement of the North American Menopause Society" (*Menopause*. 2022;29[7]:767-794. doi: 10.1097/GME .0000000000002028), with the consensus being that for healthy people born female younger than sixty, and within ten years of menopause onset, the benefits of hormone therapy outweigh the risks. This update was a significant rewrite of their prior recommendation, which said that MHT was recommended only for severe symptoms and at the lowest dose for the shortest time.

In 2020, **the American Heart Association** published "Menopause Transition and Cardiovascular Disease Risk: Implications for Timing of Early Prevention: A Scientific Statement from the American Heart Association" (*Circulation*. 2020;142[25]:e506-e532. doi:10.1161/CIR.0000000000000912). This statement acknowledged the accelerated increase in cardiovascular risk brought about by the menopausal transition and emphasized the importance of early intervention strategies to help reduce this risk. The findings noted that those who are treated with hormone therapy along with a comprehensive nutrition and lifestyle approach have lower cardiovascular risks and less likelihood of negative disease outcomes.

The United States Food and Drug Administration has approved MHT to treat four conditions associated with menopause:

1. *Vasomotor symptoms:* includes hot flashes, night sweats, heart palpitations, and sleep disturbances

2. *Bone loss:* includes weakening bones and osteoporosis

3. *Premature hypoestrogenism (estrogen deficiency):* as a result of menopause or premature menopause resulting from surgery such as oophorectomy (with or without hysterectomy), or radiation or chemotherapy

4. *Genitourinary symptoms:* includes frequent urination, burning with urination, recurrent urinary tract infections, vaginal dryness, pain with intercourse

Additionally, research has shown that hormone therapy can help improve and relieve symptoms related to the following conditions:

- SARCOPENIA (DECREASED MUSCLE MASS): Related to aging, a decrease in estrogen production, and the transition to menopause.

- COGNITION: When initiated immediately after hysterectomy with bilateral oophorectomy, estrogen therapy may provide some cognitive benefit.

- SKIN AND HAIR CONDITIONS: Includes thinning hair and skin, increased bruising, loss of skin elasticity.

- JOINT PAIN: Women participating in several studies have reported less joint pain or stiffness with hormone therapy compared with placebo.

- DIABETES: While not FDA approved for treatment of type 2 diabetes, MHT in otherwise healthy women with preexisting type 2 diabetes may improve glycemic control when used to manage menopause symptoms.

- DEPRESSION: While not FDA approved for the treatment of depression, estrogen-based therapies may complement clinical response to antidepressants in midlife and older women when prescribed to treat menopausal symptoms.

The Menopause Symptom Scoring Sheet
(THE GREENE SCALE)

Along with the updated MHT info above, you might also want to complete this Greene Scale questionnaire in preparation for an appointment with a menopausal healthcare provider.

Score each symptom 1 for mild, 2 for moderate, 3 for severe, and 0 if you do not have that particular symptom.

A score of 15 or over usually indicates that estrogen deficiency is likely contributing to your symptoms, and in my practice this means we begin the discussion of therapy immediately. Scores of 20–50 are common in symptomatic women, and with adequate treatment tailored to you, your score should reduce to 10 or under in three to six months.

SYMPTOM	SCORE
Hot Flashes	_____
Lightheaded Feelings	_____
Headaches	_____
Irritability	_____
Depression	_____
Unloved Feelings	_____
Anxiety	_____
Mood Changes	_____
Sleeplessness	_____
Unusual Tiredness	_____
Backache	_____
Joint Pain	_____
Muscle Pain	_____
New Facial Hair	_____
Dry Skin	_____
Crawling Feelings Under the Skin	_____
Less Sexual Feelings	_____
Dry Vagina	_____
Uncomfortable Intercourse	_____
Urinary Frequency	_____
TOTAL	_____

*Adapted from Greene JG. Constructing a standard climacteric standard. Maturitas 1998;29:25-31.

Hot Flash Diary/ Symptom Journal

I highly recommend that you start keeping a symptom journal of any noticeable changes to your health. Use the space below to make note of any new aches and pains, increases in fatigue, gastrointestinal issues, differences in hair or skin, weight gain or loss, mental health or memory challenges, and so on. Be as detailed as you can—your doctor will want to know how long you've been experiencing the symptoms and if they've become more or less severe. If you're not into paper and pen, keep these kinds of notes in your phone's notes app!

DATE | SYMPTOMS

DATE | SYMPTOMS

Selected References

CHAPTER 1

Chen EH, Shofer FS, Dean AJ, et al. Gender disparity in analgesic treatment of emergency department patients with acute abdominal pain. *Academic Emergency Medicine.* 2008;15(5):414-418. doi: 10.1111/j.1553-2712.2008.00100.x.

Christianson MS, Ducie JA, Altman K, Khafagy AM, Shen W. Menopause education: needs assessment of American obstetrics and gynecology residents. *Menopause.* 2013;20(11):1120-1125. doi: 10.1097/GME.0b013e31828ced7f.

Dorr B. Contributor: in the misdiagnosis of menopause, what needs to change? AJMC.com. September 14, 2022. https://www.ajmc.com/view/contributor-in-the-misdiagnosis-of-menopause-what-needs-to-change-. Accessed November 20, 2023.

Eyster KM. The estrogen receptors: an overview from different perspectives. *Methods in Molecular Biology.* 2016;1366:1-10. doi: 10.1007/978-1-4939-3127-9_1.

Farquhar CM, Sadler L, Harvey SA, Stewart AW. The association of hysterectomy and menopause: a prospective cohort study. *BJOG: An International Journal of Obstetrics and Gynaecology.* 2005;112(7):956-962. doi: 10.1111/j.1471-0528.2005.00696.x.

Hill K. The demography of menopause. *Maturitas.* 1996;23(2):113-127. doi: 10.1016/0378-5122(95)00968-x.

Kling JM, MacLaughlin KL, Schnatz PF, et al. Menopause management knowledge in postgraduate family medicine, internal medicine, and obstetrics and gynecology residents: a cross-sectional survey. *Mayo Clinic Proceedings.* 2019;94(2):242-253. doi: 10.1016/j.mayocp.2018.08.033.

Lee P, Le Saux M, Siegel R, et al. Racial and ethnic disparities in the management of acute pain in US emergency departments: meta-analysis and systematic review. *American Journal of Emergency Medicine.* 2019;37(9):1770-1777. doi: 10.1016/j.ajem.2019.06.014.

O'Neill S, Eden J. The pathophysiology of menopausal symptoms. *Obstetrics, Gynecology and Reproductive Medicine.* 2017; 27(10):303-310. doi: 10.1016/j.ogrm.2017.07.002.

Richardson MK, Coslov N, Woods NF. Seeking health care for perimenopausal symptoms: observations from the Women Living Better Survey. *Journal of Women's Health* (Larchmont). 2023;32(4):434-444. doi: 10.1089/jwh.2022.0230.

Samulowitz A, Gremyr I, Eriksson E, Hensing H. "Brave men" and "emotional women": a theory-guided literature review on gender bias in health care and gendered norms towards patients with chronic pain. *Pain Research and Management*. 2018;2018:6358624. doi: 10.1155/2018/6358624.

Shetty SA, Chandini S, Fernandes SL, Safeekh AT. Hysteria: a historical perspective. *Archives of Medicine and Health Sciences*. 2020;8(2):312-315. doi: 10.4103/amhs.amhs_220_20.

Sözen T, Özışık L, Başaran NÇ. An overview and management of osteoporosis. *European Journal of Rheumatology*. 2017;4(1):46-56. doi: 10.5152/eurjrheum.2016.048.

Tasca C, Rapetti M, Carta MG, Fadda B. Women and hysteria in the history of mental health. *Clinical Practice and Epidemiology in Mental Health*. 2012;8:110-119. doi: 10.2174/1745017901208010110.

Watkins A. Reevaluating the grandmother hypothesis. *History and Philosophy of the Life Sciences*. 2021;43:103. doi: 10.1007/s40656-021-00455-x.

Wolff J. "Doctors don't know how to treat menopause symptoms." *AARP magazine*. July 20, 2018. https://www.aarp.org/health/conditions-treatments/info-2018/menopause-symptoms-doctors-relief-treatment.html. Accessed November 20, 2023.

CHAPTER 2

Cagnacci A, Venier M. The controversial history of hormone replacement therapy. *Medicina* (Kaunas). 2019;55(9):602. doi: 10.3390/medicina55090602.

Hersh AL, Stefanick ML, Stafford RS. National use of postmenopausal hormone therapy: annual trends and response to recent evidence. *JAMA*. 2004;291(1):47-53. doi: 10.1001/jama.291.1.47.

Kohn GE, Rodriguez KM, Hotaling J, Pastuszak AW. The history of estrogen therapy. *Sexual Medicine Reviews*. 2019;7(3):416-421. doi: 10.1016/j.sxmr.2019.03.006.

Pollycove R, Naftolin F, Simon JA. The evolutionary origin and significance of menopause. *Menopause*. 2011;18(3):336-342. doi: 10.1097/gme.0b013e3181ed957a.

Singh A, Kaur S, Walia I. A historical perspective on menopause and menopausal age. *Bulletin of the Indian Institute of History of Medicine Hyderabad*. 2002;32(2):121-135.

Smith DC, Prentice R, Thompson DJ, Herrmann WL. Association of exogenous estrogen and endometrial carcinoma. *New England Journal of Medicine*. 1975;293(23):1164-1167. doi: 10.1056/NEJM197512042932302.

Smith K. Women's health research lacks funding—in a series of charts. *Nature*. 2023;617(7959):28-29. doi: 10.1038/d41586-023-01475-2.

Stefanick ML. Estrogens and progestins: background and history, trends in use, and guidelines and regimens approved by the US Food and Drug Administration. *American Journal of Medicine*. 2005;118(suppl 12B):64-73. doi: 10.1016/j.amjmed.2005.09.059.

Woods J, Warner E. The history of estrogen. *menoPAUSE* blog. February 2016. Obstetrics and Gynecology, University of Rochester Medical Center. https://www.urmc.rochester.edu/ob-gyn/ur-medicine-menopause-and-womens-health/menopause-blog/february-2016/the-history-of-estrogen.aspx. Accessed November 2, 2023.

Wren B. The history and politics of menopause. In: Panay N, Briggs P, Kovacs G, eds. *Managing the Menopause: 21st Century Solutions.* Cambridge: Cambridge University Press; 2015:20-28. doi: 10.1017/CBO9781316091821.005.

CHAPTER 3

American College of Obstetricians and Gynecologists. Hormone therapy and heart disease. Committee Opinion No. 565. *Obstetrics and Gynecology.* 2013;121:1407-1410.

Brown S. Shock, terror and controversy: how the media reacted to the Women's Health Initiative. *Climacteric.* 2012;15(3):275-280. doi: 10.3109/13697137.2012.660048.

El Khoudary SR, Aggarwal B, Beckie TM, et al. Menopause transition and cardiovascular disease risk: implications for timing of early prevention: a scientific statement from the American Heart Association. *Circulation.* 2020;142(25):e506-e532. doi: 10.1161/CIR.0000000000000912.

Hodis HN, Mack WJ. Menopausal hormone replacement therapy and reduction of all-cause mortality and cardiovascular disease: it is about time and timing. *Cancer Journal.* 2022;28(3):208-223. doi: 10.1097/PPO.0000000000000591.

Hodis HN, Mack WJ, Henderson VW, et al. Vascular effects of early versus late postmenopausal treatment with estradiol. *New England Journal of Medicine.* 2016;374(13):1221-1231. doi: 10.1056/NEJMoa1505241.

MacLennan AH. HRT: a reappraisal of the risks and benefits. *Medical Journal of Australia.* 2007;186(12):643-646. doi: 10.5694/j.1326-5377.2007.tb01084.x.

Manson JE, Chlebowski RT, Stefanick ML, et al. Menopausal hormone therapy and health outcomes during the intervention and extended poststopping phases of the Women's Health Initiative randomized trials. *JAMA.* 2013;310(13):1353-1368. doi: 10.1001/jama.2013.278040.

North American Menopause Society. Advisory Panel. The 2022 hormone therapy position statement of the North American Menopause Society. *Menopause.* 2022;29(7):767-794. doi: 10.1097/GME.0000000000002028.

Sarrel PM, Njike VY, Vinante V, Katz DL. The mortality toll of estrogen avoidance: an analysis of excess deaths among hysterectomized women aged 50 to 59 years. *American Journal of Public Health.* 2013;103(9):1583-1588. doi: 10.2105/AJPH.2013.301295.

Stefanick ML, Anderson GL, Margolis KL, et al. Effects of conjugated equine estrogens on breast cancer and mammography screening in postmenopausal women with hysterectomy. *JAMA*. 2006;295(14):1647-1657. doi: 10.1001/jama.295.14 .1647.

Sturmberg JP, Pond DC. Impacts on clinical decision making: changing hormone therapy management after the WHI. *Australian Family Physician*. 2009;38(4):249-251, 253-255. PMID: 19350076.

Writing Group for the Women's Health Initiative Investigators. Risks and benefits of estrogen plus progestin in healthy postmenopausal women: principal results from the Women's Health Initiative Randomized Controlled Trial. *JAMA*. 2002;288(3):321-333. doi: 10.1001/jama.288.3.321.

Xiangyan R, Mueck AO. Optimizing menopausal hormone therapy: for treatment and prevention, menstrual regulation, and reduction of possible risks. *Global Health Journal*. 2022;6(2):61-69. doi: 10.1016/j.glohj.2022.03.003.

CHAPTER 4

Burden L. Menopause symptoms: women are leaving workforce for little-talked-about reason. Bloomberg.com. June 18, 2021. https://www.bloomberg.com/news/articles/2021-06-18/women-are-leaving-the-workforce-for-a-little-talked-about-reason?embedded-checkout=true. Accessed November 20, 2023.

Castrillon C. Why it's time to address menopause in the workplace. *Forbes*. March 22, 2023. https://www.forbes.com/sites/carolinecastrillon/2023/03/22/why-its-time-to-address-menopause-in-the-workplace/?sh=32d717a11f72&utm _source=newsletter&utm_medium=email&utm_campaign=forbeswomen&cdl-cid=5fdca243b52f2e83d719194b. Accessed November 20, 2023.

H.R.8774. 117th Congress (2021-2022): Menopause Research Act of 2022. Accessed November 2, 2023. https://www.congress.gov/bill/117th-congress/house -bill/8774?s=1&r=13.

Landi H. Menopause care is still a largely untapped market. Here's why investors and startups should dive in. Fierce Healthcare. June 28, 2023. https://www .fiercehealthcare.com/health-tech/menopause-care-market-remains-largely -untapped-heres-why-investors-and-startups-should. Accessed December 2, 2023.

Landry DA, Yakubovich E, Cook DP, Fasih S, Upham J, Vanderhyden BC. Metformin prevents age-associated ovarian fibrosis by modulating the immune landscape in female mice. *Science Advances*. 2022;8(35):eabq1475. doi: 10.1126/sciadv.abq1475.

Mosconi L, Berti V, Quinn C, et al. Sex differences in Alzheimer risk: brain imaging of endocrine vs chronologic aging. *Neurology*. 2017;89(13):1382-1390. doi: 10.1212/WNL.0000000000004425.

Robinton D. Funding women's health research can impact the economy by

$150 billion. Fast Company. March 21, 2023. https://www.fastcompany.com/90868245/global-economic-impact-of-ignoring-this-aspect-of-womens-health-is-150-billion-we-can-do-better. Accessed November 20, 2023.

Saleh RNM, Hornberger M, Ritchie CW, Minihane AM. Hormone replacement therapy is associated with improved cognition and larger brain volumes in at-risk APOE4 women: results from the European Prevention of Alzheimer's Disease (EPAD) cohort. *Alzheimer's Research and Therapy.* 2023;15(1):10. doi: 10.1186/s13195-022-01121-5.

A study of menopause in the workplace. *Health Hub* blog. February 19, 2019. Forth. https://www.forthwithlife.co.uk/blog/menopause-in-the-workplace/. Accessed November 20, 2023.

Tang WY, Grothe D, Keshishian A, Morgenstern D, Haider S. Pharmacoeconomic and associated cost savings among women who were prescribed systemic conjugated estrogens therapy compared with those without menopausal therapy. *Menopause.* 2018;25(5):493-499. doi: 10.1097/GME.0000000000001028.

Temkin SM, Barr E, Moore H, Caviston JP, Regensteiner JG, Clayton JA. Chronic conditions in women: the development of a National Institutes of Health framework. *BMC Women's Health.* 2023;23(1):162. doi: 10.1186/s12905-023-02319-x.

Women's health: end the disparity in funding. *Nature.* 2023;617(8). doi: 10.1038/d41586-023-01472-5.

CHAPTER 5

Avis NE, Crawford SL, Greendale G, et al. Duration of menopausal vasomotor symptoms over the menopause transition. *JAMA Internal Medicine.* 2015;175(4):531-539. doi: 10.1001/jamainternmed.2014.8063.

Bae H, Lunetta KL, Murabito JM, et al. Genetic associations with age of menopause in familial longevity. *Menopause.* 2019;26(10):1204-1212. doi: 10.1097/GME.0000000000001367.

Colditz GA, Willett WC, Stampfer MJ, Rosner B, Speizer FE, Hennekens CH. Menopause and the risk of coronary heart disease in women. *New England Journal of Medicine.* 1987;316(18):1105-10. doi: 10.1056/NEJM198704303161801.

Common misdiagnoses. The Menopause Charity. October 21, 2021. https://www.themenopausecharity.org/2021/10/21/common-misdiagnoses/. Accessed November 20, 2023.

Delamater L, Santoro N. Management of the perimenopause. *Clinical Obstetrics and Gynecology.* 2018;61(3):419-432. doi: 10.1097/GRF.0000000000000389.

Ebong IA, Wilson MD, Appiah D, et al. Relationship between age at menopause, obesity, and incident heart failure: the Atherosclerosis Risk in Communities study. *Journal of the American Heart Association.* 2022;11(8):e024461. doi: 10.1161/JAHA.121.024461.

Farquhar CM, Sadler L, Harvey SA, Stewart AW. The association of hysterectomy and menopause: a prospective cohort study. *BJOG: An International Journal of Obstetrics and Gynaecology*. 2005;112(7):956-962. doi: 10.1111/j.1471-0528.2005 .00696.x.

Faubion SS, Kuhle CL, Shuster LT, Rocca WA. Long-term health consequences of premature or early menopause and considerations for management. *Climacteric*. 2015;18(4):483-491. doi: 10.3109/13697137.2015.1020484.

Foster H, Hagan J, Brooks-Gunn J, Garcia J. Association between intergenerational violence exposure and maternal age of menopause. *Menopause*. 2022;29(3):284-292. doi: 10.1097/GME.0000000000001923.

Gold EB. The timing of the age at which natural menopause occurs. *Obstetrics and Gynecology Clinics of North America*. 2011;38(3):425-440. doi: 10.1016/j.ogc .2011.05.002.

Gottschalk MS, Eskild A, Hofvind S, Bjelland EK. The relation of number of child-births with age at natural menopause: a population study of 310147 women in Norway. *Human Reproduction*. 2022;37(2):333-340. doi: 10.1093/humrep/ deab246.

Hall JE. Endocrinology of the menopause. *Endocrinology and Metabolism Clinics of North America*. 2015;44(3):485-496. doi: 10.1016/j.ecl.2015.05.010.

Kok H, van Asselt K, van der Schouw Y, et al. Heart disease risk determines meno-pausal age rather than the reverse. *Journal of the American College of Cardiology*. 2006;47(10):1976-1983. doi: 10.1016/j.jacc.2005.12.066.

Langton CR, Whitcomb BW, Purdue-Smithe AC, et al. Association of oral contra-ceptives and tubal ligation with risk of early natural menopause. *Human Repro-duction*. 2021;36(7):1989-1998. doi: 10.1093/humrep/deab054.

Li S, Ma L, Huang H, et al. Loss of muscle mass in women with premature ovarian insufficiency as compared with healthy controls. *Menopause*. 2023;30(2):122-127. doi: 10.1097/GME.0000000000002120.

Mishra GD, Pandeya N, Dobson AJ, et al. Early menarche, nulliparity and the risk for premature and early natural menopause. *Human Reproduction*. 2017;32(3):679-686. doi: 10.1093/humrep/dew350.

Newson L, Lewis R. Delayed diagnosis and treatment of menopause is wasting NHS appointments and resources. Paper presented at: the Royal College of Gen-eral Practitioners Annual Conference; 2021; London.

Parente RC, Faerstein E, Celeste RK, Werneck GL. The relationship between smoking and age at the menopause: a systematic review. *Maturitas*. 2008;61:287-298. doi: 10.1016/j.maturitas.2008.09.021.

Rosendahl M, Simonsen MK, Kjer JJ. The influence of unilateral oophorectomy on the age of menopause. *Climacteric*. 2017;20(6):540-544. doi: 10.1080/13697137 .2017.1369512.

Sarnowski C, Kavousi M, Isaacs S, et al. Genetic variants associated with earlier age at menopause increase the risk of cardiovascular events in women. *Menopause.* 2018;25(4):451-457.

Secoşan C, Balint O, Pirtea L, Grigoraş D, Bălulescu L, Ilina R. Surgically induced menopause: a practical review of literature. *Medicina* (Kaunas). 2019;55(8):482. doi: 10.3390/medicina55080482.

Shadyab AH, Macera CA, Shaffer RA, et al. Ages at menarche and menopause and reproductive lifespan as predictors of exceptional longevity in women: the Women's Health Initiative. *Menopause.* 2017;24(1):35-44. doi: 10.1097/GME .0000000000000710.

Shared decision-making. National Learning Consortium. December 2013. https:// www.healthit.gov/sites/default/files/nlc_shared_decision_making_fact_sheet .pdf. Accessed November 2, 2023.

CHAPTER 6

Abildgaard J, Tingstedt J, Zhao Y, et al. Increased systemic inflammation and altered distribution of T-cell subsets in postmenopausal women. *PLoS One.* 2020;15(6):e0235174. doi: 10.1371/journal.pone.0235174.

Bermingham KM, Linenberg I, Hall WL, et al. Menopause is associated with postprandial metabolism, metabolic health and lifestyle: the ZOE PREDICT study. *EBioMedicine.* 2022;85:104303. doi: 10.1016/j.ebiom.2022.104303.

Brinton RD, Yao J, Yin F, Mack WJ, Cadenas E. Perimenopause as a neurological transition state. *Nature Reviews Endocrinology.* 2015;11(7):393-405. doi: 10.1038 /nrendo.2015.82.

Buckinx F, Aubertin-Leheudre M. Sarcopenia in menopausal women: current perspectives. *International Journal of Women's Health.* 2022;14:805-819. doi: 10 .2147/IJWH.S340537.

Cheng CH, Chen LR, Chen KH. Osteoporosis due to hormone imbalance: an overview of the effects of estrogen deficiency and glucocorticoid overuse on bone turnover. *International Journal of Molecular Sciences.* 2022;23(3):1376. doi: 10.3390/ijms23031376.

Cui W, Zhao L. The influence of 17β-estradiol plus norethisterone acetate treatment on markers of glucose and insulin metabolism in women: a systematic review and meta-analysis of randomized controlled trials. *Frontiers in Endocrinology* (Lausanne). 2023;14:1137406. doi: 10.3389/fendo.2023.1137406.

Dam V, van der Schouw YT, Onland-Moret NC, et al. Association of menopausal characteristics and risk of coronary heart disease: a pan-European case-cohort analysis. *International Journal of Epidemiology.* 2019;48(4):1275-1285. doi:10 .1093/ije/dyz016.

De Paoli M, Zakharia A, Werstuck GH. The role of estrogen in insulin resistance: a review of clinical and preclinical data. *American Journal of Pathology.* 2021;191(9):1490-1498. doi: 10.1016/j.ajpath.2021.05.011.

Geraci A, Calvani R, Ferri E, Marzetti E, Arosio B, Cesari M. Sarcopenia and menopause: the role of estradiol. *Frontiers in Endocrinology* (Lausanne). 2021;12:682012. doi: 10.3389/fendo.2021.682012.

Giannos P, Prokopidis K, Candow DG, et al. Shorter sleep duration is associated with greater visceral fat mass in US adults: findings from NHANES, 2011–2014. *Sleep Medicine.* 2023;105:78-84. doi: 10.1016/j.sleep.2023.03.013.

Gibson CJ, Shiozawa A, Epstein AJ, Han W, Mancuso S. Association between vasomotor symptom frequency and weight gain in the Study of Women's Health Across the Nation. *Menopause.* 2023;30(7):709-716. doi: 10.1097/GME .0000000000002198.

Gosset A, Pouillès JM, Trémollieres F. Menopausal hormone therapy for the management of osteoporosis. *Best Practice and Research Clinical Endocrinology and Metabolism.* 2021;35(6):101551. doi: 10.1016/j.beem.2021.101551.

Herrera AY, Mather M. Actions and interactions of estradiol and glucocorticoids in cognition and the brain: implications for aging women. *Neuroscience and Biobehavioral Reviews.* 2015;55:36-52. doi: 10.1016/j.neubiorev.2015.04 .005.

Hettchen M, von Stengel S, Kohl M, et al. Changes in menopausal risk factors in early postmenopausal osteopenic women after 13 months of high-intensity exercise: the randomized controlled ACTLIFE-RCT. *Clinical Interventions in Aging.* 2021;16:83-96. doi: 10.2147/CIA.S283177.

Hou Q, Guan Y, Yu W, et al. Associations between obesity and cognitive impairment in the Chinese elderly: an observational study. *Clinical Interventions in Aging.* 2019;14:367-373. doi: 10.2147/CIA.S192050.

Juppi HK, Sipilä S, Fachada V, et al. Total and regional body adiposity increases during menopause: evidence from a follow-up study. *Aging Cell.* 2022;21(6):e13621. doi: 10.1111/acel.13621.

Katsoulis M, Benetou V, Karapetyan T, et al. Excess mortality after hip fracture in elderly persons from Europe and the USA: the CHANCES project. *Journal of Internal Medicine.* 2017;281(3):300-310. doi: 10.1111/joim.12586.

Ko S-H, Kim H-S. Menopause-associated lipid metabolic disorders and foods beneficial for postmenopausal women. *Nutrients.* 2020;12(1):202. https://doi.org/10 .3390/nu12010202.

Kodoth V, Scaccia S, Aggarwal B. Adverse changes in body composition during the menopausal transition and relation to cardiovascular risk: a contemporary review. *Women's Health Reports* (New Rochelle). 2022;3(1):573-581. doi: 10.1089/ whr.2021.0119.

Maki PM, Jaff NG. (2022) Brain fog in menopause: a health-care professional's guide for decision-making and counseling on cognition. *Climacteric.* 2022;25:6:570-578. doi: 10.1080/13697137.2022.2122792.

Marsh ML, Oliveira MN, Vieira-Potter VJ. Adipocyte metabolism and health after the menopause: the role of exercise. *Nutrients.* 2023;15(2):444. doi: 10.3390/nu15020444.

Mauvais-Jarvis F, Manson JE, Stevenson JC, Fonseca VA. Menopausal hormone therapy and type 2 diabetes prevention: evidence, mechanisms, and clinical implications. *Endocrine Reviews.* 2017;38(3):173-188. doi: 10.1210/er.2016-1146.

McCarthy M, Raval AP. The peri-menopause in a woman's life: a systemic inflammatory phase that enables later neurodegenerative disease. *Journal of Neuroinflammation.* 2020;17(317). doi: 10.1186/s12974-020-01998-9.

Menopause and bone loss. Endocrine Society. August 22, 2023. https://www.endocrine.org/patient-engagement/endocrine-library/menopause-and-bone-loss. Accessed November 21, 2023.

Miller AP, Chen YF, Xing D, Feng W, Oparil S. Hormone replacement therapy and inflammation: interactions in cardiovascular disease. *Hypertension.* 2003;42(4):657-663. doi: 10.1161/01.HYP.0000085560.02979.0C.

Panula J, Pihlajamäki H, Mattila VM, et al. Mortality and cause of death in hip fracture patients aged 65 or older: a population-based study. *BMC Musculoskeletal Disorders.* 2011;12:105. doi: 10.1186/1471-2474-12-105.

Papadakis GE, Hans D, Rodriguez EG, et al. Menopausal hormone therapy is associated with reduced total and visceral adiposity: the OsteoLaus cohort. *Journal of Clinical Endocrinology and Metabolism.* 2018;103(5):1948-1957. doi: 10.1210/jc.2017-02449.

Pertesi S, Coughlan G, Puthusseryppady V, Morris E, Hornberger M. Menopause, cognition and dementia: a review. *Post Reproductive Health.* 2019;25(4):200-206. doi: 10.1177/2053369119883485.

Porchia LM, Vazquez-Marroquin G, Ochoa-Précoma R, Pérez-Fuentes R, Gonzalez-Mejia ME. Probiotics' effect on visceral and subcutaneous adipose tissue: a systematic review of randomized controlled trials. *European Journal of Clinical Nutrition.* 2022;76(12):1646-1656. doi: 10.1038/s41430-022-01135-0.

Pu D, Tan R, Yu Q, Wu J. Metabolic syndrome in menopause and associated factors: a meta-analysis. *Climacteric.* 2017;20(6):583-591. doi: 10.1080/13697137.2017.1386649.

Santoro N, Randolph JF Jr. Reproductive hormones and the menopause transition. *Obstetrics and Gynecology Clinics of North America.* 2011;38(3):455-466. doi: 10.1016/j.ogc.2011.05.004.

Schelbaum E, Loughlin L, Jett S, et al. Association of reproductive history with brain MRI biomarkers of dementia risk in midlife. *Neurology.* 2021;97(23):e2328-e2339. doi: 10.1212/WNL.0000000000012941.

Shanmugan S, Epperson CN. Estrogen and the prefrontal cortex: towards a new understanding of estrogen's effects on executive functions in the menopause transition. *Human Brain Mapping.* 2014;35(3):847-865. doi: 10.1002/hbm.22218.

Williamson L. Hormones are key in brain health differences between men and women. American Heart Association. February 1, 2021. https://www.heart.org/en/news/2021/02/01/hormones-are-key-in-brain-health-differences-between-men-and-women. Accessed August 4, 2021.

Yasui T, Maegawa M, Tomita J, et al. Changes in serum cytokine concentrations during the menopausal transition. *Maturitas.* 2007;56(4):396-403. doi: 10.1016/j.maturitas.2006.11.002.

Zeydan B, Atkinson EJ, Weis DM, et al. Reproductive history and progressive multiple sclerosis risk in women. *Brain Communications.* 2020;2(2):fcaa185. doi: 10.1093/braincomms/fcaa185.

Zhang H, Ma K, Li RM. et al. Association between testosterone levels and bone mineral density in females aged 40–60 years from NHANES 2011–2016. *Science Reports.* 2022 Sep 30;12(1):16426. https://doi.org/10.1038/s41598-022-21008-7

CHAPTER 7

American College of Obstetricians and Gynecologists. Postmenopausal estrogen therapy: route of administration and risk of venous thromboembolism. Committee Opinion No. 556. *Obstetrics and Gynecology.* 2013;121:887-890.

Bianchi VE, Bresciani E, Meanti R, Rizzi L, Omeljaniuk RJ, Torsello A. The role of androgens in women's health and wellbeing. *Pharmacological Research.* 2021;171:105758. doi: 10.1016/j.phrs.2021.105758.

Cold S, Cold F, Jensen MB, Cronin-Fenton D, Christiansen P, Ejlertsen B. Systemic or vaginal hormone therapy after early breast cancer: a Danish observational cohort study. *Journal of the National Cancer Institute.* 2022;114(10):1347-1354. doi: 10.1093/jnci/djac112.

DiSilvestro JB, Haddad J, Robison K, et al. Barriers to hormone therapy following prophylactic bilateral salpingo-oophorectomy in BRCA1/2 mutation carriers. *Menopause.* 2023;30(7):732-737. doi: 10.1097/GME.0000000000002201.

FDA takes action against compounded menopause hormone therapy drugs. Fierce Biotech, January 10, 2008. https://www.fiercebiotech.com/biotech/fda-takes-action-against-compounded-menopause-hormone-therapy-drugs. Accessed November 21, 2023.

Hamoda H, Panay N, Pedder H, Arya R, Savvas M. The British Menopause Society and Women's Health Concern 2020 recommendations on hormone replacement therapy in menopausal women. *Post Reproductive Health.* 2020;26(4):181-209. doi: 10.1177/2053369120957514.

Huber D, Seitz S, Kast K, Emons G, Ortmann O. Hormone replacement therapy in

BRCA mutation carriers and risk of ovarian, endometrial, and breast cancer: a systematic review. *Journal of Cancer Research and Clinical Oncology.* 2021;147(7):2035-2045. doi: 10.1007/s00432-021-03629-z.

North American Menopause Society. Advisory Panel. The 2022 hormone therapy position statement of the North American Menopause Society. *Menopause.* 2022;29(7):767-794. doi: 10.1097/GME.0000000000002028.

Pinkerton JV. Concerns about compounded bioidentical menopausal hormone therapy. *Cancer Journal.* 2022;28(3):241-245. doi: 10.1097/PPO .0000000000000597.

Tang J, Chen LR, Chen KH. The utilization of dehydroepiandrosterone as a sexual hormone precursor in premenopausal and postmenopausal women: an over-view. *Pharmaceuticals* (Basel). 2021;15(1):46. doi: 10.3390/ph15010046.

CHAPTER 8

Brigden ML. Clinical utility of the erythrocyte sedimentation rate. *American Family Physician.* 1999;60(5):1443-1450.

Dwyer JB, Aftab A, Radhakrishnan R, et al. Hormonal Treatments for Major Depressive Disorder: State of the Art [published correction appears in *American Journal of Psychiatry.* 2020 Jul 1;177(7):642] [published correction appears in *American Journal of Psychiatry.*2020 Oct 1;177(10):1009]. *American Journal of Psychiatry.* 2020;177(8):686-705. doi:10.1176/appi.ajp.2020.19080848.

Evron JM, Herman WH, McEwen LN. Changes in screening practices for prediabetes and diabetes since the recommendation for hemoglobin A1c testing [published correction appears in *Diabetes Care.* 2020;43(9):2323]. *Diabetes Care.* 2019;42(4):576-584. doi: 10.2337/dc17-1726.

Freeman AM, Rai M, Morando DW. Anemia screening. [Updated July 25, 2023]. In: StatPearls [Internet]. Treasure Island, FL: StatPearls Publishing; 2023. https://www.ncbi.nlm.nih.gov/books/NBK499905/. Accessed November 21, 2023.

Gervais NJ, Au A, Almey A, Duchesne A, Gravelsins L, Brown A, Reuben R, Baker-Sullivan E, Schwartz DH, Evans K, Bernardini MQ, Eisen A, Meschino WS, Foulkes WD, Hampson E, Einstein G. Cognitive markers of dementia risk in middle-aged women with bilateral salpingo-oophorectomy prior to menopause. *Neurobiol Aging.* 2020 Oct;94:1-6. doi: 10.1016/j.neurobiolaging.2020.04 .019. Epub 2020 Apr 29. PMID: 32497876.

Greene JG. Constructing a standard climacteric scale. *Maturitas.* 1998;29(1):25-31. doi: 10.1016/s0378-5122(98)00025-5.

Greene JG. A factor analytic study of climacteric symptoms. *Journal of Psychosomatic Research.* 1976;20:425-430.

Heaney RP. Vitamin D in health and disease. *Clinical Journal of the American Society of Nephrology.* 2008;3(5):1535-41. doi: 10.2215/CJN.01160308.

Mauvais-Jarvis F, Manson JE, Stevenson JC, Fonseca VA. Menopausal hormone therapy and type 2 diabetes prevention: evidence, mechanisms, and clinical implications. *Endocr Rev.* 2017 Jun 1;38(3):173-188. https://doi.org/10.1210/er.2016-1146.

Maxfield L, Shukla S, Crane JS. Zinc deficiency. [Updated June 28, 2023]. In: StatPearls [Internet]. Treasure Island, FL: StatPearls Publishing; 2023. https://www.ncbi.nlm.nih.gov/books/NBK493231/. Accessed November 21, 2023.

Mei Y, Williams JS, Webb EK, Shea AK, MacDonald MJ, Al-Khazraji BK. Roles of hormone replacement therapy and menopause on osteoarthritis and cardiovascular disease outcomes: a narrative review. *Front Rehabil Sci.* 2022 Mar 28;3:825147. doi: 10.3389/fresc.2022.825147. PMID: 36189062; PMCID: PMC9397736.

Onambélé-Pearson GL, Tomlinson DJ, Morse CI, Degens H. A prolonged hiatus in postmenopausal HRT, does not nullify the therapy's positive impact on ageing related sarcopenia. *PLoS One.* 2021 May 5;16(5):e0250813. doi: 10.1371/journal.pone.0250813. PMID: 33951065; PMCID: PMC8099084.

Parva NR, Tadepalli S, Singh P, et al. Prevalence of vitamin D deficiency and associated risk factors in the US population (2011–2012). *Cureus.* 2018;10(6):e2741. doi: 10.7759/cureus.2741.

Prasad M, Sara J, Widmer RJ, Lennon R, Lerman LO, Lerman A. Triglyceride and triglyceride/ HDL (high density lipoprotein) ratio predict major adverse cardiovascular outcomes in women with non-obstructive coronary artery disease. *Journal of the American Heart Association.* 2019;8(9):e009442. doi: 10.1161/JAHA.118.009442.

Ridker PM. High-sensitivity C-reactive protein and cardiovascular risk: rationale for screening and primary prevention. *American Journal of Cardiology.* 2003;92(4B):17K-22K. doi: 10.1016/s0002-9149(03)00774-4.

Schwalfenberg GK, Genuis SJ. The importance of magnesium in clinical healthcare. *Scientifica* (Cairo). 2017;2017:4179326. doi: 10.1155/2017/4179326.

Watson J, Round A, Hamilton W. Raised inflammatory markers. *BMJ.* 2012;344:e454. doi: 10.1136/bmj.e454.

CHAPTER 9

Cowan S, Dordevic A, Sinclair AJ, Truby H, Sood S, Gibson S. Investigating the efficacy and feasibility of using a whole-of-diet approach to lower circulating levels of C-reactive protein in postmenopausal women: a mixed methods pilot study. *Menopause.* 2023;30(7):738-749. doi: 10.1097/GME.0000000000002188.

Hao S, Tan S, Li J, et al. Dietary and exercise interventions for perimenopausal women: a health status impact study. *Frontiers in Nutrition.* 2022;8:752500. doi: 10.3389/fnut.2021.752500.

Hao S, Tan S, Li J, et al. The effect of diet and exercise on climacteric symptomatol-
ogy. *Asia Pacific Journal of Clinical Nutrition*. 2022;31(3):362-370. doi: 10.6133/
apjcn.202209_31(3).0004.

Mishra N, Mishra VN, Devanshi. Exercise beyond menopause: dos and don'ts.
Journal of Midlife Health. 2011;2(2):51-56. doi: 10.4103/0976-7800.92524.

Olson EJ. Can lack of sleep make you sick? Mayo Clinic, November 28, 2018.
https://www.mayoclinic.org/diseases-conditions/insomnia/expert-answers/lack
-of-sleep/faq-20057757. Accessed November 21, 2023.

CHAPTER 10

Abe RAM, Masroor A, Khorochkov A, et al. The role of vitamins in non-alcoholic
fatty liver disease: a systematic review. *Cureus*. 2021;13(8):e16855. doi: 10.7759/
cureus.16855.

Abildgaard J, Ploug T, Al-Saoudi E, et al. Changes in abdominal subcutaneous adipose tissue phenotype following menopause is associated with increased visceral
fat mass. *Scientific Reports*. 2021;11:14750. https://doi.org/10.1038/s41598-021
-94189-2.

Agostini D, Zeppa Donati S, Lucertini F, et al. Muscle and bone health in postmenopausal women: role of protein and vitamin D supplementation combined
with exercise training. *Nutrients*. 2018;10(8):1103. doi: 10.3390/nu10081103.

Alcohol and the immune system: what you should know. Gateway Foundation,
December 16, 2022. https://www.gatewayfoundation.org/addiction-blog/alcohol
-immune-system/. Accessed September 8, 2023.

Angum F, Khan T, Kaler J, Siddiqui L, Hussain A. The prevalence of autoimmune
disorders in women: a narrative review. *Cureus*. 2020;12(5):e8094. doi: 10.7759/
cureus.8094.

Arab A, Rafie N, Amani R, Shirani F. The role of magnesium in sleep health: a systematic review of available literature. *Biological Trace Element Research*.
2023;201(1):121-128. doi: 10.1007/s12011-022-03162-1.

Baan EJ, de Roos EW, Engelkes M, et al. Characterization of asthma by age of
onset: a multi-database cohort study. *Journal of Allergy and Clinical Immunology
in Practice*. 2022;10(7):1825-1834.e8. doi: 10.1016/j.jaip.2022.03.019.

Baker FC, Lampio L, Saaresranta T, Polo-Kantola P. Sleep and sleep disorders in
the menopausal transition. *Sleep Medicine Clinics*. 2018;13(3):443-456. doi: 10
.1016/j.jsmc.2018.04.011.

Barnard ND, Kahleova H, Holtz DN, et al. A dietary intervention for vasomotor
symptoms of menopause: a randomized, controlled trial. *Menopause*.
2023;30(1):80-87. doi: 10.1097/GME.0000000000002080.

Behrman S, Crockett C. Severe mental illness and the perimenopause. BJPsych
Bulletin. 2023:1-7. doi:10.1192/bjb.2023.89.

Beaumont M, Goodrich JK, Jackson MA, et al. Heritable components of the human fecal microbiome are associated with visceral fat. *Genome Biology.* 2016;17(1):189. doi: 10.1186/s13059-016-1052-7.

Boneva RS, Lin J-MS, Unger ER. Early menopause and other gynecologic risk indicators for chronic fatigue syndrome in women. *Menopause.* 2015;22(8):826-834. doi: 10.1097/GME.0000000000000411.

Boneva RS, Maloney EM, Lin JM, et al. Gynecological history in chronic fatigue syndrome: a population-based case-control study. *Journal of Women's Health (Larchmont).* 2011;20(1):21-28. doi: 10.1089/jwh.2009.1900.

Calvani R, Picca A, Coelho-Júnior HJ, Tosato M, Marzetti E, Landi F. Diet for the prevention and management of sarcopenia. *Metabolism.* 2023;146:155637. doi: 10.1016/j.metabol.2023.155637.

Carpenter JS, Sheng Y, Pike C, et al. Correlates of palpitations during menopause: a scoping review. *Women's Health* (London). 2022;18:17455057221112267. doi: 10 .1177/17455057221112267.

Chacko SA, Song Y, Manson JE, et al. Serum 25-hydroxyvitamin D concentrations in relation to cardiometabolic risk factors and metabolic syndrome in post-menopausal women. *American Journal of Clinical Nutrition.* 2011;94(1):209-217. doi: 10.3945/ajcn.110.010272.

Chen C, Gong X, Yang X, et al. The roles of estrogen and estrogen receptors in gastrointestinal disease. *Oncology Letters.* 2019;18(6):5673-5680. doi: 10.3892/ol .2019.10983.

Chen HC, Chung CH, Chen VCF, Wang YC, Chien WC. Hormone replacement therapy decreases the risk of tinnitus in menopausal women: a nationwide study. *Oncotarget.* 2018;9(28):19807-19816. doi: 10.18632/oncotarget.24452.

Chen Y, Zhang Y, Zhao G, et al. Difference in leukocyte composition between women before and after menopausal age, and distinct sexual dimorphism. *PLoS One.* 2016;11(9):e0162953. doi: 10.1371/journal.pone.0162953.

Chessa MA, Iorizzo M, Richert B, et al. Pathogenesis, clinical signs and treatment recommendations in brittle nails: a review [published correction appears in *Dermatology and Therapy* (Heidelberg). 2020;10(1):231-232]. *Dermatology and Therapy* (Heidelberg). 2020;10(1):15-27. doi: 10.1007/s13555-019-00338-x.

Chilibeck PD, Candow DG, Landeryou T, Kaviani M, Paus-Jenssen L. Effects of creatine and resistance training on bone health in postmenopausal women. *Medicine and Science in Sports and Exercise.* 2015;47(8):1587-1595. doi: 10.1249 /MSS.0000000000000571.

Chimenos-Kustner E, Marques-Soares MS. Burning mouth and saliva. *Medicina Oral.* 2002;7(4):244-253. PMID: 12134125.

Cicero AFG, Colletti A, Bellentani S. Nutraceutical approach to non-alcoholic fatty liver disease (NAFLD): the available clinical evidence. *Nutrients.* 2018;10(9):1153. doi: 10.3390/nu10091153.

Davis SR. Androgen therapy in women, beyond libido. *Climacteric.* 2013;16 Suppl 1:18-24. doi:10.3109/13697137.2013.801736.

da Costa Hime LFC, Carvalho Lopes CM, Roa CL, et al. Is there a beneficial effect of gamma-linolenic acid supplementation on body fat in postmenopausal hypertensive women? a prospective randomized double-blind placebo-controlled trial. *Menopause.* 2021;28(6):699-705. doi: 10.1097/GME.0000000000001740.

Decandia D, Landolfo E, Sacchetti S, Gelfo F, Petrosini L, Cutuli D. 2022. n-3 PUFA improve emotion and cognition during menopause: a systematic review. *Nutrients.* 2022;14(9):1982. doi: 10.3390/nu14091982.

Deecher DC, Dorries K. Understanding the pathophysiology of vasomotor symptoms (hot flushes and night sweats) that occur in perimenopause, menopause, and postmenopause life stages. *Archives of Women's Mental Health.* 2007;10(6):247-257. doi: 10.1007/s00737-007-0209-5.

de Koning L, Merchant AT, Pogue J, Anand SS. Waist circumference and waist-to-hip ratio as predictors of cardiovascular events: meta-regression analysis of prospective studies. *European Heart Journal.* 2007;28(7):850-856. doi: 10.1093/eurheartj/ehm026.

Desai MK, Brinton RD. Autoimmune disease in women: endocrine transition and risk across the lifespan. *Frontiers in Endocrinology* (Lausanne). 2019;10:265. doi: 10.3389/fendo.2019.00265.

DiStefano JK. NAFLD and NASH in postmenopausal women: implications for diagnosis and treatment. *Endocrinology.* 2020;161(10):bqaa134. doi: 10.1210/endocr/bqaa134.

Doshi SB, Agarwal A. The role of oxidative stress in menopause. *Journal of Midlife Health.* 2013;4(3):140-146. doi: 10.4103/0976-7800.118990.

Dutt P, Chaudhary S, Kumar P. Oral health and menopause: a comprehensive review on current knowledge and associated dental management. *Annals of Medical and Health Science Research.* 2013;3(3):320-323. doi: 10.4103/2141-9248 .117926.

Elffers TW, de Mutsert R, Lamb HJ, et al. Body fat distribution, in particular visceral fat, is associated with cardiometabolic risk factors in obese women. *PLoS One.* 2017;12(9):e0185403. doi: 10.1371/journal.pone.0185403.

Epstein JB, Marcoe JH. Topical application of capsaicin for treatment of oral neuropathic pain and trigeminal neuralgia. *Oral Surgery, Oral Medicine, Oral Pathology, and Oral Radiology.* 1994;77(2):135-140. doi: 10.1016/0030 -4220(94)90275-5.

Florentino GS, Cotrim HP, Vilar CP, Florentino AV, Guimarães GM, Barreto VS.

Nonalcoholic fatty liver disease in menopausal women. *Arquivos de Gastroenterologia*. 2013;50(3):180-185. doi: 10.1590/S0004-28032013000200032.

Fong C, Alesi S, Mousa A, et al. Efficacy and safety of nutrient supplements for glycaemic control and insulin resistance in type 2 diabetes: an umbrella review and hierarchical evidence synthesis. *Nutrients*. 2022;14(11):2295. doi: 10.3390/nu14112295.

Forabosco A, Criscuolo M, Coukos G, et al. Efficacy of hormone replacement therapy in postmenopausal women with oral discomfort. *Oral Surgery, Oral Medicine, Oral Pathology, and Oral Radiology*. 1992;73(5):570-574. doi: 10.1016 0030-4220(92)90100-5.

Galhardo APM, Mukai MK, Baracat MCP, et al. Does temporomandibular disorder correlate with menopausal symptoms? *Menopause*. 2022;29(6):728-733. doi: 10.1097/GME.0000000000001962.

Gava G, Orsili I, Alvisi S, Mancini I, Seracchioli R, Meriggiola MC. Cognition, mood and sleep in menopausal transition: the role of menopause hormone therapy. *Medicina* (Kaunas). 2019;55(10):668. doi: 10.3390/medicina55100668.

Geller SE, Studee L. Botanical and dietary supplements for mood and anxiety in menopausal women. *Menopause*. 2007;14(3 Pt 1):541-549. doi: 10.1097/01.gme .0000236934.43701.c5.

Gibson CJ, Shiozawa A, Epstein AJ, Han W, Mancuso S. Association between vasomotor symptom frequency and weight gain in the Study of Women's Health Across the Nation. *Menopause*. 2023;30(7):709-716. doi: 10.1097/GME .0000000000002198.

Gregersen I, Høibraaten E, Holven KB, et al. Effect of hormone replacement therapy on atherogenic lipid profile in postmenopausal women. *Thrombosis Research*. 2019;184:1-7. doi: 10.1016/j.thromres.2019.10.005.

Gremeau-Richard C, Woda A, Navez ML, et al. Topical clonazepam in stomatodynia: a randomised placebo-controlled study. *Pain*. 2004;108(1-2):51-57. doi: 10.1016/j.pain.2003.12.002.

Gualano B, Macedo AR, Alves CR, et al. Creatine supplementation and resistance training in vulnerable older women: a randomized double-blind placebo-controlled clinical trial. *Experimental Gerontology*. 2014;53:7-15. doi: 10.1016/j. exger.2014.02.003.

Hansen ESH, Aasbjerg K, Moeller AL, Gade EJ, Torp-Pedersen C, Backer V. Hormone replacement therapy and development of new asthma. *Chest*. 2021;160(1):45-52. doi: 10.1016/j.chest.2021.01.054.

Hatzichristou D, Kirana PS, Banner L, et al. Diagnosing sexual dysfunction in men and women: sexual history taking and the role of symptom scales and questionnaires. *Journal of Sexual Medicine*. 2016;13(8):1166-1182.

Hatzichristou D, Rosen RC, Broderick G, et al. Clinical evaluation and management strategy for sexual dysfunction in men and women. *Journal of Sexual Medicine.* 2004;1(1):49-57.

Heckmann SM, Kirchner E, Grushka M, Wichmann MG, Hummel T. A double-blind study on clonazepam in patients with burning mouth syndrome. *Laryngoscope.* 2012;122(4):813-816. doi: 10.1002/lary.22490.

Herrera AY, Hodis HN, Mack WJ, Mather M. Estradiol therapy after menopause mitigates effects of stress on cortisol and working memory. *Journal of Clinical Endocrinology and Metabolism.* 2017;102(12):4457-4466. doi: 10.1210/jc.2017 -00825.

Herrera AY, Mather M. Actions and interactions of estradiol and glucocorticoids in cognition and the brain: implications for aging women. *Neuroscience and Biobehavioral Reviews.* 2015;55:36-52. doi: 10.1016/j.neubiorev.2015.04.005.

Hunter GR, Singh H, Carter SJ, Bryan DR, Fisher G. Sarcopenia and its implications for metabolic health. *Journal of Obesity.* 2019;2019:8031705. doi: 10.1155/ 2019/8031705.

Hyon JY, Han SB. Dry eye disease and vitamins: a narrative literature review. *Applied Sciences.* 2022;12(9):4567. doi: 10.3390/app12094567.

Illescas-Montes R, Melguizo-Rodríguez L, Ruiz C, Costela-Ruiz VJ. Vitamin D and autoimmune diseases. *Life Sciences.* 2019;233:116744. doi: 10.1016/j.lfs.2019 .116744.

Institute of Medicine (US) and National Research Council (US) Committee on the Framework for Evaluating the Safety of Dietary Supplements. *Dietary Supplements: A Framework for Evaluating Safety.* Washington, DC: National Academies Press (US); 2005. Appendix K, Prototype Focused Monograph: Review of Antiandrogenic Risks of Saw Palmetto Ingestion by Women. https://www.ncbi .nlm.nih.gov/books/NBK216069/. Accessed November 21, 2023.

Janssen I, Powell LH, Kazlauskaite R, Dugan SA. Testosterone and visceral fat in midlife women: the Study of Women's Health Across the Nation (SWAN) fat patterning study. *Obesity* (Silver Spring). 2010;18(3):604-610. doi: 10.1038/oby .2009.251.

Jaroenlapnopparat A, Charoenngam N, Ponvilawan B, Mariano M, Thongpiya J, Yingchoncharoen P. Menopause is associated with increased prevalence of non-alcoholic fatty liver disease: a systematic review and meta-analysis. *Menopause.* 2023;30(3):348-354. doi: 10.1097/GME.0000000000002133.

Jeong SH. Benign paroxysmal positional vertigo risk factors unique to perimenopausal women. *Frontiers in Neurology.* 2020;11:589605. doi: 10.3389/fneur.2020 .589605.

Jett S, Malviya N, Schelbaum E, et al. Endogenous and exogenous estrogen exposures: how women's reproductive health can drive brain aging and inform Alzheimer's prevention. *Frontiers in Aging Neuroscience.* 2022;14:831807. doi: 10 .3389/fnagi.2022.831807.

Kendall AC, Pilkington SM, Wray JR, et al. Menopause induces changes to the stratum corneum ceramide profile, which are prevented by hormone replacement therapy. *Science Reports.* 2022;12:21715. doi: 10.1038/s41598-022-26095-0.

Kendrick M. Should women be offered cholesterol lowering drugs to prevent cardiovascular disease? No. *BMJ.* 2007;334(7601):983. doi: 10.1136/bmj.39202 .397488.AD.

Khadilkar SS. Musculoskeletal disorders and menopause. *Journal of Obstetrics and Gynaecology of India.* 2019;69(2):99-103. doi: 10.1007/s13224-019-01213-7.

Khunger N, Mehrotra K. Menopausal acne: challenges and solutions. *International Journal of Women's Health.* 2019;11:555-567. doi: 10.2147/IJWH.S174292.

Kim MS, Choi YJ, Lee YH. Visceral fat measured by computed tomography and the risk of breast cancer. *Translational Cancer Research.* 2019;8(5):1939-1949. doi: 10.21037/tcr.2019.09.16.

Kim SE, Min JS, Lee S, et al. Different effects of menopausal hormone therapy on non-alcoholic fatty liver disease based on the route of estrogen administration. *Science Reports.* 2023;13:15461. https://doi.org/10.1038/s41598-023-42788-6.

Kingsberg SA, Faubion SS. Clinical management of hypoactive sexual desire disorder in postmenopausal women. *Menopause.* 2022;29(9):1083-1085. doi: 10 .1097/GME.0000000000002049.

Klempel MC, Kroeger CM, Bhutani S, Trepanowski JF, Varady KA. Intermittent fasting combined with calorie restriction is effective for weight loss and cardioprotection in obese women. *Nutrition Journal.* 2012;11:98. doi: 10.1186/1475 -2891-11-98.

Ko J, Park YM. Menopause and the loss of skeletal muscle mass in women. *Iranian Journal of Public Health.* 2021;50(2):413-414. doi: 10.18502/ijph.v50i2.5362.

Kodoth V, Scaccia S, Aggarwal B. Adverse changes in body composition during the menopausal transition and relation to cardiovascular risk: a contemporary review. *Women's Health Reports* (New Rochelle). 2022;3(1):573-581. doi: 10.1089/ whr.2021.0119.

Koppen LM, Whitaker A, Rosene A, Beckett RD. Efficacy of berberine alone and in combination for the treatment of hyperlipidemia: a systematic review. *Journal of Evidence Based Complementary Alternative Medicine.* 2017;22(4):956-968. doi: 10.1177/2156587216687695.

Kroenke CH, Caan BJ, Stefanick ML, et al. Effects of a dietary intervention and weight change on vasomotor symptoms in the Women's Health Initiative. *Menopause.* 2012;19(9):980-988. doi: 10.1097/gme.0b013e31824f606e.

Krüger M, Obst A, Ittermann T, et al. Menopause is associated with obstructive sleep apnea in a population-based sample from Mecklenburg-Western Pomerania, Germany. *Journal of Clinical Medicine.* 2023;12(6):2101. doi: 10.3390/jcm12062101.

Lakhan SE, Vieira KF. Nutritional therapies for mental disorders. *Nutrition Journal.* 2008;7:2. doi: 10.1186/1475-2891-7-2.

Lambeau KV, McRorie JW Jr. Fiber supplements and clinically proven health benefits: how to recognize and recommend an effective fiber therapy. *Journal of the American Association of Nurse Practitioners.* 2017;29(4):216-223. doi: 10.1002/2327-6924.12447.

Leon-Ferre RA, Novotny P, Faubion SS, et al. A randomized, double-blind, placebo-controlled trial of oxybutynin for hot flashes: ACCRU study SC-1603. Paper presented at: the 2018 San Antonio Breast Cancer Symposium; San Antonio, TX; December 7, 2018. Abstract GS6-02.

Lephart ED, Naftolin F. Menopause and the skin: old favorites and new innovations in cosmeceuticals for estrogen-deficient skin. *Dermatology and Therapy* (Heidelberg). 2021;11(1):53-69. doi: 10.1007/s13555-020-00468-7.

Leslie MA, Cohen DJA, Liddle DM, et al. A review of the effect of omega-3 polyunsaturated fatty acids on blood triacylglycerol levels in normolipidemic and borderline hyperlipidemic individuals. *Lipids in Health and Disease.* 2015;14:53. doi: 10.1186/s12944-015-0049-7.

Lim S, Moon JH, Shin CM, Jeong D, Kim B. Effect of *Lactobacillus sakei*, a probiotic derived from kimchi, on body fat in Koreans with obesity: a randomized controlled study. *Endocrinology and Metabolism* (Seoul). 2020;35(2):425-434. doi: 10.3803/EnM.2020.35.2.425.

Lin CM, Davidson TM, Ancoli-Israel S. Gender differences in obstructive sleep apnea and treatment implications. *Sleep Medicine Reviews.* 2008;12(6):481-496. doi: 10.1016/j.smrv.2007.11.003.

Liu Y, Alookaran JJ, Rhoads JM. Probiotics in autoimmune and inflammatory disorders. *Nutrients.* 2018;10(10):1537. doi: 10.3390/nu10101537.

Lu CB, Liu PF, Zhou YS, et al. Musculoskeletal pain during the menopausal transition: a systematic review and meta-analysis. *Neural Plasticity.* 2020;2020:8842110. doi: 10.1155/2020/8842110.

Lufkin EG, Wahner HW, O'Fallon WM, et al. Treatment of postmenopausal osteoporosis with transdermal estrogen. *Annals of Internal Medicine.* 1992;117(1):1-9. doi: 10.7326/0003-4819-117-1-1.

Maki PM, Jaff NG. (2022) Brain fog in menopause: a health-care professional's guide for decision-making and counseling on cognition. *Climacteric.* 2022;25(6):570-578. doi: 10.1080/13697137.2022.2122792.

Maki PM, Rubin LH, Savarese A, et al. Stellate ganglion blockade and verbal memory in midlife women: evidence from a randomized trial. *Maturitas.* 2016;92:123-129. doi: 10.1016/j.maturitas.2016.07.009.

Mannucci C, Casciaro M, Sorbara EE, et al. Nutraceuticals against oxidative stress in autoimmune disorders. *Antioxidants* (Basel). 2021;10(2):261. doi: 10.3390/antiox10020261.

Manson JE, Chlebowski RT, Stefanick ML, et al. Menopausal hormone therapy and health outcomes during the intervention and extended poststopping phases of the Women's Health Initiative randomized trials. *JAMA.* 2013;310(13):1353-1368. doi: 10.1001/jama.2013.278040.

Mao T, Huang F, Zhu X, Wei D, Chen L. (2021). Effects of dietary fiber on glycemic control and insulin sensitivity in patients with type 2 diabetes: a systematic review and meta-analysis. *Journal of Functional Foods.* 2021;82:104500. doi: 10.1016/j.jff.2021.104500.

Mitchell ES, Woods NF. Pain symptoms during the menopausal transition and early postmenopause. *Climacteric.* 2010;13(5):467-478. doi: 10.3109/13697137.2010.483025.

Momin ES, Khan AA, Kashyap T, et al. The effects of probiotics on cholesterol levels in patients with metabolic syndrome: a systematic review. *Cureus.* 2023;15(4):e37567. doi: 10.7759/cureus.37567.

Morozov S, Isakov V, Konovalova M. Fiber-enriched diet helps to control symptoms and improves esophageal motility in patients with non-erosive gastroesophageal reflux disease. *World Journal of Gastroenterology.* 2018;24(21):2291-2299. doi: 10.3748/wjg.v24.i21.2291.

Mosconi L, Berti V, Dyke J, et al. Menopause impacts human brain structure, connectivity, energy metabolism, and amyloid-beta deposition. *Science Reports.* 2021;11:10867. doi: 10.1038/s41598-021-90084-y.

Nie G, Yang X, Wang Y, et al. The effects of menopause hormone therapy on lipid profile in postmenopausal women: a systematic review and meta-analysis. *Frontiers in Pharmacology.* 2022;13:850815. doi: 10.3389/fphar.2022.850815.

North American Menopause Society. Management of osteoporosis in postmenopausal women: the 2021 position statement of the North American Menopause Society. *Menopause.* 2021;28(9):973-997. doi: 10.1097/GME.0000000000001831.

North American Menopause Society. Advisory Panel. The 2023 nonhormone therapy position statement of the North American Menopause Society. *Menopause.* 2023;30(6):573-590. doi: 10.1097/GME.0000000000002200.

Ogun OA, Büki B, Cohn ES, Janky KL, Lundberg YW. Menopause and benign paroxysmal positional vertigo. *Menopause.* 2014;21(8):886-889. doi: 10.1097/GME.0000000000000190.

Papadakis GE, Hans D, Gonzalez Rodriguez E, et al. Menopausal hormone therapy is associated with reduced total and visceral adiposity: the OsteoLaus cohort. *Journal of Clinical Endocrinology and Metabolism.* 2018;103(5):1948-1957. doi: 10.1210/jc.2017-02449.

Parish SJ, Kling JM. Testosterone use for hypoactive sexual desire disorder in post-menopausal women. *Menopause.* 2023;30(7):781-783. doi: 10.1097/GME .0000000000002190.

Park Y, Sinn DH, Kim K, et al. Associations of physical activity domains and muscle strength exercise with non-alcoholic fatty liver disease: a nation-wide cohort study. *Science Reports.* 2023;13:4724. doi: 10.1038/s41598-023-31686-6.

Pasiakos SM, Lieberman HR, Fulgoni VL 3rd. Higher-protein diets are associated with higher HDL cholesterol and lower BMI and waist circumference in US adults. *Journal of Nutrition.* 2015;145(3):605-614. doi: 10.3945/jn.114.205203.

Peters BA, Lin J, Qi Q, et al. Menopause is associated with an altered gut microbiome and estrobolome, with implications for adverse cardiometabolic risk in the Hispanic Community Health Study/Study of Latinos. *mSystems.* 2022;7(3):e0027322. doi: 10.1128/msystems.00273-22.

Peters BA, Santoro N, Kaplan RC, Qi Q. Spotlight on the gut microbiome in menopause: current insights. *International Journal of Women's Health.* 2022;14:1059-1072. doi: 10.2147/IJWH.S340491.

Proksch E, Schunck M, Zague V, Segger D, Degwert J, Oesser S. Oral intake of specific bioactive collagen peptides reduces skin wrinkles and increases dermal matrix synthesis. *Skin Pharmacology and Physiology.* 2014;27(3):113-119. doi: 10 .1159/000355523.

Robinson JL, Johnson PM, Kister K, Yin MT, Chen J, Wadhwa S. Estrogen signaling impacts temporomandibular joint and periodontal disease pathology. *Odontology.* 2020;108(2):153-165. doi: 10.1007/s10266-019-00439-1.

Sanchez M, Darimont C, Drapeau V, et al. Effect of *Lactobacillus rhamnosus* CGMCC1.3724 supplementation on weight loss and maintenance in obese men and women. *British Journal of Nutrition.* 2014;111(8):1507-1519. doi: 10.1017/ S0007114513003875.

Sardella A, Lodi G, Demarosi F, Tarozzi M, Canegallo L, Carrassi A. *Hypericum perforatum* extract in burning mouth syndrome: a randomized placebo-controlled study. *Journal of Oral Pathology and Medicine.* 2008;37(7):395-401. doi: 10.1111/j.1600-0714.2008.00663.x.

Shah SA, Tibble H, Pillinger R, et al. Hormone replacement therapy and asthma onset in menopausal women: national cohort study. *Journal of Allergy and Clinical Immunology.* 2021;147(5):1662-1670. doi: 10.1016/j.jaci.2020.11.024.

Sheng Y, Carpenter JS, Elomba CD, et al. Effect of menopausal symptom treatment options on palpitations: a systematic review. *Climacteric.* 2022;25(2):128-140. doi: 10.1080/13697137.2021.1948006.

Sheng Y, Carpenter JS, Elomba CD, et al. Review of menopausal palpitations measures. *Women's Midlife Health.* 2021;7(1):5. doi: 10.1186/s40695-021-00063-6.

Shibli F, El Mokahal A, Saleh S, Fass R. Menopause is an important risk factor for GERD and its complications in women. *American Journal of Gastroenterology.* 2021;116:S168-S169. doi: 10.14309/01.ajg.0000774008.23848.49.

Shulman LP. Transdermal hormone therapy and bone health. *Clinical Interventions in Aging.* 2008;3(1):51-54. doi: 10.2147/cia.s937.

Siddle N, Sarrel P, Whitehead M. The effect of hysterectomy on the age at ovarian failure: identification of a subgroup of women with premature loss of ovarian function and literature review. *Fertility and Sterility.* 1987;47(1):94-100. doi: 10.1016/s0015-0282(16)49942-5.

Silva TR, Spritzer PM. Skeletal muscle mass is associated with higher dietary protein intake and lower body fat in postmenopausal women: a cross-sectional study. *Menopause.* 2017;24(5):502-509. doi: 10.1097/GME.0000000000000793.

Singh A, Asif N, Singh PN, Hossain MM. Motor nerve conduction velocity in postmenopausal women with peripheral neuropathy. *Journal of Clinical and Diagnostic Research.* 2016;10(12):CC13-CC16. doi: 10.7860/JCDR/2016/23433.9004.

Stevenson J, Medical Advisory Council of the British Menopause Society. Prevention and treatment of osteoporosis in women. *Post Reproductive Health.* 2023;29(1):11-14. doi: 10.1177/20533691221139902.

Studd J. Ten reasons to be happy about hormone replacement therapy: a guide for patients. *Menopause International.* 2010;16(1):44-46. doi: 10.1258/mi.2010.010001.

Tarhuni M, Fotso MN, Gonzalez NA, et al. Estrogen's tissue-specific regulation of the SLC26A6 anion transporter reveal a phenotype of kidney stone disease in estrogen-deficient females: a systematic review. *Cureus.* 2023;15(9):e45839. doi: 10.7759/cureus.45839.

Taylor-Swanson L, Wong AE, Pincus D, et al. The dynamics of stress and fatigue across menopause: attractors, coupling, and resilience. *Menopause.* 2018;25(4):380-390. doi: 10.1097/GME.0000000000001025.

Thaung Zaw JJ, Howe PRC, Wong RHX. Long-term resveratrol supplementation improves pain perception, menopausal symptoms, and overall well-being in postmenopausal women: findings from a 24-month randomized, controlled, crossover trial. *Menopause.* 2020;28(1):40-49. doi: 10.1097/GME.0000000000001643.

Tijerina A, Barrera Y, Solis-Pérez E, et al. Nutritional risk factors associated with vasomotor symptoms in women aged 40-65 years. *Nutrients.* 2022;14(13):2587. doi: 10.3390/nu14132587.

Triebner K, Johannessen A, Puggini L, et al. Menopause as a predictor of new-onset asthma: a longitudinal northern European population study. *Journal of Al-*

lergy and Clinical Immunology. 2016;137(1):50-57.e6. doi: 10.1016/j.jaci.2015.08 .019.

Turek J, Gąsior Ł. Estrogen fluctuations during the menopausal transition are a risk factor for depressive disorders. *Pharmacology Reports.* 2023;75:32-43. https://doi.org/10.1007/s43440-022-00444-2.

Volpe A, Lucenti V, Forabosco A, et al. Oral discomfort and hormone replacement therapy in the post-menopause. *Maturitas.* 1991;13(1):1-5. doi: 10.1016/0378 -5122(91)90279-y.

Wardrop RW, Hailes J, Burger H, Reade PC. Oral discomfort at menopause. *Oral Surgery, Oral Medicine, Oral Pathology, and Oral Radiology.* 1989;67(5):535-40. doi: 10.1016/0030-4220(89)90269-7.

Waxman J, Zatzkis SM. (1986) Fibromyalgia and menopause. *Postgraduate Medicine.* 1986;80(4):165-171. doi: 10.1080/00325481.1986.11699544.

Wesström J, Ulfberg J, Nilsson S. Sleep apnea and hormone replacement therapy: a pilot study and a literature review. *Acta Obstetricia et Gynecologica Scandinavica.* 2005;84(1):54-57. doi: 10.1111/j.0001-6349.2005.00575.x.

Whalley LJ, Starr JM, Deary IJ. Diet and dementia. *Journal of the British Menopause Society.* 2004;10(3):113-117. doi: 10.1258/1362180043654575.

Wong RHX, Evans HM, Howe PRC. Resveratrol supplementation reduces pain experience by postmenopausal women. *Menopause.* 2017;24(8):916-922. doi: 10 .1097/GME.0000000000000861.

Yan H, Yang W, Zhou F, et al. Estrogen improves insulin sensitivity and suppresses gluconeogenesis via the transcription factor Foxo1. *Diabetes.* 2019;68(2):291-304. doi: 10.2337/db18-0638.

Yoo SZ, No MH, Heo JW, et al. Role of exercise in age-related sarcopenia. *Journal of Exercise Rehabilitation.* 2018;14(4):551-558. doi: 10.12965/jer.1836268.134.

Zdzieblik D, Oesser S, König D. Specific bioactive collagen peptides in osteopenia and osteoporosis: long-term observation in postmenopausal women. *Journal of Bone Metabolism.* 2021;28(3):207-213. doi: 10.11005/jbm.2021.28.3.207.

Zhang S, Hu J, Fan W, et al. Aberrant cerebral activity in early postmenopausal women: a resting-state functional magnetic resonance imaging study. *Frontiers in Cellular Neuroscience.* 2018;12:454. doi: 10.3389/fncel.2018.00454.

Zhu D, Chung HF, Dobson AJ, et al. Vasomotor menopausal symptoms and risk of cardiovascular disease: a pooled analysis of six prospective studies. *American Journal of Obstetrics and Gynecology.* 2020;223(6):898.e1-898.e16. doi: 10.1016/j .ajog.2020.06.039.

Acknowledgments

In expressing my gratitude for the incredible journey of writing *The New Menopause*, I am humbled by the unwavering support and inspiration from those who have played pivotal roles in this endeavor.

My deepest appreciation goes to my family—my rock throughout this process. To my husband, Christopher Haver; my children, Katherine Haver my moon and stars and Madeline Haver my sun; and my sister, Leah Lynn Pastor—your ceaseless encouragement, invaluable insights, and unwavering belief in my ability have been the driving forces behind this project.

In memory of my brothers in heaven—Jep, Bob, and Jude Pastor—their untimely deaths remain poignant reminders of why I embarked on this journey and have helped stay the course.

To my father in heaven, Patrick J. Pastor—a life well lived and loved. To my mother, Mary Marguerite Landry Pastor—how she has survived the unthinkable will always inspire me.

A special acknowledgment to Gretchen Lees for the incredible collaborative effort in writing this book. Your insight and friendship transformed my dry scientific prose into a coherent narrative filled with humor, intelligence, and heart.

To my agent, Heather Jackson—thank you for standing by me through the creation of two books, for being a constant sounding board, and above all, for being a wonderful friend.

I extend my gratitude to Editor Marnie Cochran and the exceptional team at Harmony Rodale, especially Jonathan Sung, for their contributions to shaping and supporting the production of this book.

A heartfelt acknowledgment to my internal team at the 'Pause Life—the incomparable Jen Pearson—without whom I would be toiling in obscurity, Jamie Hadley who manages to manage my time and every opportunity that heads my way, Margaret Walsh who represents the soul of our company, and Dawn Drogash whose organizational development skills are second to none, and to Gabi Anderson, Zach Toth, Jackie Schaiper, Kristen Lewis, Victoria Thomas, and Sara Joseph—for keeping the ship running and managing countless social media messages and emails, hundreds of thousands of students in our programs, thousands of monthly orders of our products, all while keeping me sane so I could have time to research and write.

My heartfelt appreciation to Donna Gately, my right and left hand. Thank you for calling out when I needed it and holding me accountable to the things that matter. I could not have done this without you.

To my team at Mary Claire Wellness Clinic—Joan Moss, Stacy Lord, Ciara Madigan, Kennedy Harrington, and Mary Turner—thank you for your dedication to our patients and continuous collaboration.

I am indebted to the fellow voices in the social media "Meno-verse"—an incredible group of brilliant, driven, like-minded professionals that includes: Dr. Sharon Malone, Dr. Kelly Casperson, Dr. Corinne Menn, Dr. Avrum Bluming and team at Estrogen Matters, Dr. Suzanne Gilberg-Lenz, Dr. Alicia Jackson, Tamsen Fadal, Alisa Volkman, Dr. Heather Hirsh, Dr. Lisa Mosconi, Dr. Vonda Wright, Dr. Gabrielle Lyon, Alicia Jackson, Anne Fulenwider, and Monica Molenaar. Your constant support, interest and engagement in idea-sharing, and celebration of each other's successes have been invaluable.

To my Galveston Island tribe—Heidi Seigel, Cara Koza, Pamela Gabriel, Emily Root, Dr. Erica Kelly, Dr. Lisa Farmer, Stephanie Vasut, Le Bergin, Tysh Mefferd, Amy Gaido, and Paige Cook—thank you for your unwavering friendship, your children who made my world a better place, our thousands of laughs together, and your hugs for my tears.

A special acknowledgment to my cousins (but really sisters) Marla Fowler, Lizette Thompson, and Gerryl Krilic for your never-ending love and support.

I extend my deepest gratitude to Dr. Sharon McCloskey, Dr. Kate White, Dr. Belinda Schwertner, Dr. Russel Snyder, Deb Millard, Dr. Jen Ashton, Naomi Watts, Ani Hadjinian, Amy Griffin, Brene' Brown, and Dr. Anthony (Tony) Youn, Stephannie Haver Castex, and Rosemary Haver for their contributions and influence on this journey.

And finally, to everyone who has followed and engaged with me on social media: your pursuit of insight and guidance on menopause has helped make me a better doctor and educator, and I value your trust in me as an advocate more than you know. Thank you for helping fuel my passion for research and driving my search for answers—and for being an integral part of "The New Menopause." I wrote this book for you.

Index

About the Author

DR. MARY CLAIRE HAVER is board certified in Obstetrics and Gynecology, and a Certified Menopause Specialist through The Menopause Society. She is also a Certified Culinary Medicine Specialist from Tulane University. She is a Louisiana State University Medical Center graduate and completed her Obstetrics and Gynecology residency at the University of Texas Medical Branch (UTMB). In her professional career, Dr. Haver has served as a clinical professor at UTMB and the University of Texas Health Science Center at Houston. In 2021, she opened Mary Claire Wellness, a clinic dedicated to caring for the menopausal patient. Dr. Haver has amassed more than 3.5 million followers across social media platforms by posting evidence-based guidance for women going through menopause. She lives with her husband in Galveston, Texas, and is the mother of two grown daughters.

www.thepauselife.com

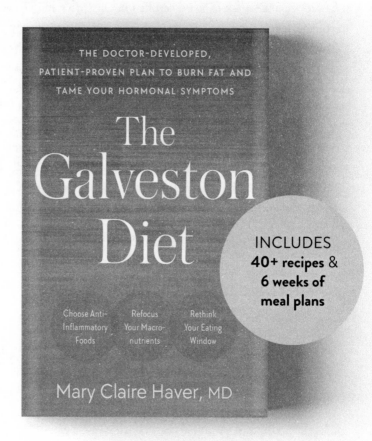